The Pennington Plan

The Pennington Plan

5 Simple Steps for Achieving Vibrant Health,
Emotional Well-Being, and Spiritual Growth

ANDREA PENNINGTON, M.D., C.AC.
with ABIGAIL PENNINGTON, M.D.

AVERY
a member of Penguin Group (USA) Inc.
New York

AVERY

Published by the Penguin Group

Penguin Group (USA) Inc., 375 Hudson Street, New York, New York 10014, USA · Penguin Group (Canada), 10 Alcorn Avenue, Toronto, Ontario, Canada M4V 3B2 (a division of Pearson Penguin Canada Inc.) · Penguin Books Ltd, 80 Strand, London WC2R 0RL, England · Penguin Ireland, 25 St Stephen's Green, Dublin 2, Ireland (a division of Penguin Books Ltd) · Penguin Group (Australia), 250 Camberwell Road, Camberwell, Victoria 3124, Australia (a division of Pearson Australia Group Pty Ltd) · Penguin Books India Pvt Ltd, 11 Community Centre, Panchsheel Park, New Delhi – 110 017, India · Penguin Group (NZ), Cnr Airborne and Rosedale Roads, Albany, Auckland 1310, New Zealand (a division of Pearson New Zealand Ltd) · Penguin Books (South Africa) (Pty) Ltd, 24 Sturdee Avenue, Rosebank, Johannesburg 2196, South Africa · Penguin Books Ltd, Registered Offices: 80 Strand, London WC2R 0RL, England

Library of Congress Cataloging-in-Publication Data

Pennington, Andrea.
The Pennington plan : 5 simple steps for achieving vibrant health, emotional well-being, and spiritual growth / Andrea Pennington with Abigail Pennington.
p. cm.
ISBN 1-58333-193-X
1. Holistic medicine. 2. Mind and body. 3. Health.
I. Pennington, Abigail. II. Title.
R733+ 2004055127
615.5—dc22

Printed in the United States of America
1 3 5 7 9 10 8 6 4 2

Book design by Aldo Sampieri

PUBLISHER'S NOTE: Neither the author(s) nor the publisher is engaged in rendering professional advice or services to the individual reader. The ideas, procedures, and suggestions in this book are not intended as a substitute for consulting a physician. All matters regarding health require medical supervision. Neither the author(s) nor the publisher shall be liable or responsible for any loss, injury, or damage allegedly arising from any information or suggestion in this book. The opinions expressed in this book represent the personal views of the author(s) and not of the publisher. Names and identifying information of the people depicted in this book have been changed to protect their privacy.

Most Avery books are available at special quantity discounts for bulk purchase for sales promotions, premiums, fund-raising, and educational needs. Special books or book excerpts also can be created to fit specific needs. For details, write Penguin Group (USA) Inc. Special Markets, 375 Hudson Street, New York, NY 10014.

ACKNOWLEDGMENTS

I would like to extend sincere thanks to the many individuals who have each offered encouragement, guidance, and support while I poured my time and passion into this project. To my mother, Dr. Abigail Pennington, contributing author and mentor, I truly appreciate your guidance. To my father, Gerald Pennington, thank you for your support in providing me with "tranquility time" in the Ruby Mountains. To John Duff, who had the vision and faith that I would produce a truly helpful guide to wellness, thank you. Noah, your love and understanding amaze and inspire me. Alexander, your insight and laughter remind me of what I already know. Thanks for repeating yourself—often. To Todd Shuster, who provided solid support and understanding as I fiercely stood my ground on the creative process, I truly value you! I send my appreciation to my editor at Avery, Dara Stewart, whose honesty was and is priceless. I am sincerely grateful for the nurturing comments, edits, and interviews conducted by Joel Segel, who succeeded at preserving the truth of my animated voice. Finally I must acknowledge the profound contribution that my patients, their families, and Life Makeover participants have offered me. You have taught me to remain open, creative, and humble. Thank you for allowing me to enrich your lives as you have mine.

CONTENTS

The Pennington Plan

Introduction

The Pennington Plan
and How to Use It

The Pennington Plan will lay out before you a clear path to wellness. This easy five-step plan will help you bring the different parts of your self—mind, body, and spirit—into balance and harmony. The impact on your health, career, relationships, and mental and emotional well-being will be immediate and far-reaching. The principles of the plan are not difficult: as you understand and absorb them, the negative thinking or bad habits that have hindered you in achieving your goals in the past will slowly but steadily begin to fade away. With sufficient desire, belief, and dedication, you will gain access to—and learn to maintain—the sense of well-being that already resides in your mind and heart.

Part One will present the belief that lies at the heart of the Pennington Plan: wellness is your natural state. Wellness, you will come to believe, is your birthright. I will explain the origin of disease, and you will discover that you never need be unwell again. Together, we will confront any doubts or skepticism you may have about this and enable you to face the dragons that have hindered your health progress in the past.

In Part Two you will begin to see your mind, body, and spirit as a single, interconnected whole. If any part of your being, especially your spirit, is not nurtured, supported, and expressed, the resulting imbalance will eventually express itself as disease. For optimal health and happiness, you must pay heed to and maintain proper balance in each. You will also learn that through your spirit you have access to enormous energy and the power to ease or possibly even erase disease. By becoming conscious of your innate personal power and by gaining more understanding of the intricate connections among these three parts of your being, you will see dramatic improvements in all areas of your life.

In Part Three we delineate the five-step plan that will help you perfect the integration and balance of spirit, mind, and body. It will not be hard to follow, and it will not involve a difficult process. The structure and guidance mechanism built into the plan will train you to live well instinctively. We will work together to define your goals, examine your motivation for attaining them, and design a realistic plan for their achievement. We will explore ways to maintain your motivation and enthusiasm until you once again make wellness your permanent state of residence. However, your success will depend upon the strength of your commitment to your goals and to the plan. You may need to change your behavior and mindset. You may need to reach deep within your soul for strength. There are no magic spells, potions, or pills to put you into a perfect state of health. But you do possess the tools; they lie within. I will show you how a five-step plan can work miracles. But *you* will have to "work it." By diligently following the plan, you *will* experience success. You will achieve the optimal well-being that you had long forgotten was possible but that is, in fact, your natural state.

As each chapter builds on the one before, I suggest that you read this book, at your own pace, from beginning to end. You will find that this will help you assimilate and implement new information logically, leading you to recognize your natural ownership of power and knowledge—the keys to your wellness destiny.

Each of the plan's five steps draws on strengths inherent in each part of your being: your spirit, mind, and body. You will quickly find that these five steps can be applied to all aspects of your life for total life fulfillment. I have included lessons and suggested exercises that will help you solidify these life-changing concepts in your mind. I suggest that you dedicate a journal or notebook to these exercises for full benefit of the process. Carry your journal with you at all times to record your inspirations and thoughts. Reflect upon these to help set the concepts in your mind and to erase the faulty beliefs that may be keeping you trapped in sickness.

Finally, at the end of each chapter, you will find affirmations that will aid in further imprinting the new concepts into your subconscious. They help replace old, negative thought patterns and empower you to achieve success. Come back to them often. I suggest that you create your own affirmations as well—affirmations that are specific to your individual goals.

Words spoken with conviction or strong emotion can hurt or heal you. For instance, three little words like "I love you" can send you into rapture. Praise can boost your mood and confidence. Destructive comments and criticism can cause anxiety and depression just as easily, especially if you believe them to be based in truth. Mood is more than just an abstract notion: our moods are directly linked to the chemistry of our bodies. Mood changes cause our brains to respond by pouring out chemicals that carry signals throughout the rest of the brain and the body. So though they may not break bones, cruel words actually *can* hurt us, by sending chemical shockwaves all through the body.

This is why it is so important that you replace self-defeating internal beliefs with positive affirmations. Beliefs like "I've been fat all of my life. I'll always be fat. My whole family is fat" become self-fulfilling prophecies. Your mind can do nothing but ensure that these statements remain true, because you have so installed them in your very being.

On the other hand, you have the power to replace your fears with hope. Instead of waiting to hear words from others that could uplift you, you can say them to yourself. That is the purpose of each chapter's affirmations. Commit these affirmations to memory. Repeat them several times each day, until they seep into your consciousness and begin to influence every organ in your body. Doing so not only can raise your mood, but also can affect your health. You can stimulate changes in the very cells of your body that have the power to improve your health and stimulate vitality.

One caveat is that your mind must believe what your mouth is saying. So if the affirmations written at the end of the chapters are not quite what you need to hear, write your own. Use words from your goal description as affirmations. If you are working on losing weight, then repeat every day to yourself, "I am achieving my goal weight. I am becoming slender, healthy, and active. I am satisfied with eating smaller portions of food. I enjoy getting more physical activity." If you talk to yourself like this and visualize your goal, you will transmit images into the deep center of your brain. If you couple this with the active steps that you will devise using this plan, your brain will begin to respond by changing your metabolism and channeling energy into the production of your goal. Your neurotransmitters and hormones, whose complex interplay produces your moods, will respond to your convictions.

The time to start creating greater health and well-being and enjoying life in a whole new way is *now*. The time to put an end to self-defeating practices and tend the garden within is *now*. Ready to enjoy better health and vitality? Let's get started!

Understanding Wellness

CHAPTER 1

Wellness Is Your Birthright— and You Have the Power to Reclaim It

We all want to feel well: not just "not sick," but truly *well* in the deepest sense of the word. But what does wellness really mean?

Wellness is a joyful state in which spirit, mind, and body are vibrant and active. From a state of wellness you are able to fully participate in life with energy, enthusiasm, and optimism. Wellness creates joie de vivre. It wraps everything that it encounters with joy. It gives us the confidence, the desire, and the ability to enjoy life fully. Achieving a true state of wellness turns life's simplest pleasures into causes for celebration. Wellness produces a sense of purpose—a feeling that we are born for a reason. Only from this state can we truly love and accept ourselves and contribute to the well-being of those around us.

Wellness does not necessarily imply the absence of disease. It is something you can choose to enjoy once again no matter what your health status. Despite the presence of an illness or psychological condition, you are entitled to and *can* enjoy wellness. By creating harmony among mind, spirit, and body, you can embrace this glorious state and thrive *despite* illness or distress. Whatever your social or economic level may be, wellness is yours to reclaim—now.

Too many of us today find ourselves in poor physical, emotional, and spiritual states, dead-end relationships, and uninspiring careers. Depression, illness, and disability sometimes seem more the norm than the exception. With the often-frenetic pace of our lifestyles, most of us are unable to focus our attention and efforts in a sustained or meaningful way to improve our health and well-being. Others are not even aware that greater health and well-being are possible. We overlook or deny the root cause of our suffering and instead try to ease the pain with drugs, food, or destructive behaviors. This is truly unfortunate, as these detrimental activities put us on the slippery slope to even worse health. Worst of all is that most people feel powerless to improve their condition, whereas the opposite is true: *The power to improve your life and put yourself back on the road to wellness lies within you.*

What do we humans need to truly thrive? We need adequate food, clothing, and shelter, of course. But taking care of our immediate physical needs is not enough. We also need activity, laughter, self-expression, excitement. We need even deeper things as well: love, spiritual connectedness, self-knowledge, wisdom. Together, these things nurture and sustain our whole being—body, mind, and spirit. We need them all if we expect to live a well-adjusted life.

Healing begins within. In order to create and maintain wellness, you must take care of your whole self, giving proper care and attention not only to your body but to your spirit and mind as well. The mind is of particular importance because it often imposes limitations and false ideas of weakness that can lead to and perpetuate illness. The physical body is an outward expression of your inner composition. Negative emotions, physically destructive behaviors, addictive substances, poor nutrition, lack of exercise, stifled dreams, stressful living conditions, sleep deprivation—all these contribute to blocking your natural vitality and robust spirit. When you are full of toxic substances and toxic emotions, your body may respond by manifesting pain, disease, and disability. Usually "disease" means that the body is not performing as it should. Here we will use the term *disease* to describe any illness or imbalance of the spirit, mind, or body—a state of being at odds, unbalanced, uncontrolled. Most of the dis-ease we see today is reversible and preventable. You can reclaim the condition of wellness and ultimately put an end to needless suffering and despair.

Restoring Balance, Reviving Resilience

Before you will enjoy lasting results in the outer world, you must restore proper balance to your inner world. Though you may have forgotten how to achieve it, you have the inborn capacity for such balance.

My training in pediatrics and early years as a doctor confirmed that wellness is a state we naturally occupy before our thinking becomes cluttered by outside influence and conditioning. During surgical rotations in my medical training, it was remarkable to me that within six to eight hours after having his appendix removed, a five-year-old child would be begging to visit the playroom, while a fifty-year-old man would plead for more pain medication and a note to excuse him from his job for an additional week. Certainly physical differences were at work, but by and large the difference lay in the mind.

Children naturally embody a spirit of resilience and vigor. As a child you were always exploring fresh sensations and looking for new challenges. Balancing mind, body, and spirit was second nature to you. Your body was constantly in motion. Your mind was always curious, always seeking new information, always asking why. Your spirit and passion were constantly being expressed in games and activities. As children we do not possess any limiting information that suggests that we are incapable of doing anything we set our minds to. We believe we can turn cardboard boxes into rocket ships, and we do. We believe we can become a doctor *and* an astronaut. We can do anything that our hearts desire—and it is all such fun. We don't worry about the mistakes we make. We do not assume that when things hurt, break, or fall apart, we have been personally wronged, robbed, or punished. Children have no restrictive belief systems, except those installed through the influence of someone else. Unless and until we learn otherwise, we believe that we can conquer all. We believe that anything and *everything* is still possible for us.

Taking care of sick children taught me that whether or not illness defeats us is often a matter of personal decision. A sick child does not identify with the pain or illness. She does not become attached to it or allow it to define her. She will simply pick herself up and begin moving about again as soon as possible. She may ask, "Why is this happening to me?" but, despite her infirmity, she will soon be planning the next adventure, tea party, or expedition. I often saw children with one leg in a cast hopping about and playing rambunctiously: wasting time and energy lamenting their lack of mobility never seemed to occur to them. Even children with chronic or terminal illnesses or physical disabilities will often tell magical stories to anyone who will listen. They express their inner liveliness by drawing and painting pictures. They plan their futures.

I believe that this tendency toward vitality is inborn, that the resilient condition of childhood is our natural state of being and only becomes inactive through the conditioning of the mind. I also believe that the capacity for this healthy disposition continues to exist within us today. The conditioning and programming of your mind by experience, parents, peers, the media, and the rest of society have stripped away your innocence and resilience. Fortunately, you can remove the negative, limiting influences that have been programmed into your mind and reclaim wellness. It takes a concerted effort, but it can be done. Repeating the affirmations and doing the lessons in this book will begin to melt that conditioning away. You can choose to believe in and draw upon the healing power that lies within you, not just to survive but to thrive. We will explore the mind's profound influence on all of the body's organs and systems in Chapter 3. For now it is enough to know that your thoughts critically affect your physical health and overall well-being.

Embracing Spirit, Mind, and Body

To thrive as children naturally do, even in the face of illness, we must learn first to recognize the proper function of each aspect of our being, then to balance and integrate them. This is the foundation of our plan for reclaiming wellness. Tapping into your spiritual nature, taking charge of your thought processes, and nourishing your body will create both outward physical joy and a rich internal environment of psychological and spiritual well-being. A physical deficiency or learning disability may cause you to rely more heavily on one part of your being or another, but for absolute function, each part of your makeup must be given the proper attention and respect. You simply cannot thrive if any aspect of your being is neglected or mistreated—or overemphasized. You cannot experience wellness or enjoy life when you deny who you really are. In the here and now, adequate attention must be given to physical and emotional pain, but for absolute relief of illness and suffering, a true cure is needed. You must deal with the root cause of your distress. Embracing our whole nature allows us to tap into our reason for being, our destiny. This starts with healing the mind and giving permission to spirit to reenter into the experience of life. I use the term *spirit*, in general, to refer to that untouchable, unseen part of ourselves that is connected to the energy of all life. It is a vital force, an essence, and can be interpreted in many ways. The story of one of our patients, Sonya, illustrates this concept well.

Sonya's Story

Sonya is a thirty-four-year-old woman who for several years suffered with irritable bowel syndrome, anxiety disorder, and insomnia. For the last few years, she was under extreme pressure at an unfulfilling job with coworkers she described as "negative." Amid several interpersonal clashes, and being fed up with feeling unappreciated and put upon, Sonya decided to leave her job and sought our advice to get her life and health back on track. I began our first session by conducting a stress assessment and taking a detailed history of her past and present illnesses. I asked her to tell me more about her current work environment. I also asked about her childhood and upbringing. Here is what she told me.

As a child, Sonya had been heavily involved with the arts. She danced, played piano, and performed in school plays. She even attended a performing arts high school and was enrolled in the gifted and talented program throughout her school career. When Sonya entered her senior year of high school, a guidance counselor at school explained that to "make it in the world," she would need to choose a profession in business, engineering, or computers. He suggested she begin preparing for a college education in one of those fields. Her parents echoed the guidance counselor, telling their daughter that she needed to choose a profitable career that would allow her to become self-sufficient. With no encouragement to pursue a career in the performing arts, Sonya decided upon computer science and attended the local state college.

Sonya realized early on that her classmates were "not like her." She felt that their interests, demeanor, and spirit were totally unlike her own. They had no interest in music, theater, or any aspect of the arts; they seemed content to study mathematics for hours on end. Though Sonya hated the coursework, she studied diligently, believing that her success depended upon her performance in her chosen career path. Far from being happy, she felt depressed. She was not expressing her creativity or any of her passions. She was not dancing or playing piano. She didn't attend plays. She told me that she no longer considered these things to be worthwhile.

When Sonya graduated, she joined a large consulting firm in a computer-related position. She survived, but did not thrive, in that company, for six years. She later moved to another consulting firm where she had been employed for the past nine years. During the first few years, Sonya really tried to "get ahead." She worked long hours, took on extra projects, and did everything to make her boss look good. Unfortunately, despite all her hard work, she was passed over for promotions. Sonya believed her supervisor was intimidated by her strong-willed personality. She sought the advice of friends. Quit complaining, they told her. You have a good job. You get a great paycheck, with a 401(k) and benefits. Don't make waves; just suck it up. Sonya decided to play it safe. She suppressed her disappointment and continued doing what she could to get along with her boss.

Finally, she reached a point where things were really explosive and confrontational at work. None of her attempts at reconciliation had helped. Convinced she was a victim of discrimination, she brought suit against the company. In the months that followed, Sonya suffered with terrible constipation, insomnia, and anxiety attacks. She was plagued with doubt and frustration about her future. She knew she had to leave the job regardless of what sort of settlement might come. But where would she go next? She hated the career that she had trained for and felt desperate and paralyzed. She worried that no real opportunities were available to her.

Sonya explained to me that she could no longer take the "safe" route with the career she had mistakenly chosen at the behest of a well-intentioned yet misguided guidance counselor. She felt as if she had no one to turn to, no one to listen to or understand her side, and no one to help her work through her frustration. She could no longer confide in her friends because they only saw the job title, the money, and the security. Plagued by her intestinal discomfort, anxiety, and insomnia, she began to shut down. She withdrew from friends and family, stopped exercising, and found herself sleeping excessively in the afternoons on her days off. She felt that she truly needed our help.

There is no doubt in my mind that Sonya's constipation was brought on by internalizing her stress and denying the expression of her artistic passions. The paralysis she felt in her mind and spirit had been translated into intestinal paralysis—constipation. Sonya also displayed classic signs of depression, though she didn't recognize them as such. She had sleep disturbances, she withdrew from normally pleasurable activities, and she felt numb and hopeless.

I explained to Sonya that I completely understood her situation, as it closely resembled my own. I, too, had been a performer as a child: an actor, a singer, a dancer. The world of make-believe was always mine. At the same time, I always wanted to follow in my mother's footsteps and become a doctor. I really wanted to help people, and I felt that was the best way to make a contribution to the world. All the way through pre-med, I continued to sing and do theater, but medical school forced me to withdraw from my artistic pursuits, just as Sonya's consulting job was doing. I couldn't sing; I couldn't perform. Without the things that gave me that inner joy and sent my spirit soaring, I became profoundly depressed. It was only much later that I found ways to integrate the different sides of myself. So when Sonya came in, I knew what she was going through. I knew she was discovering, as I had, that *de*nied ex*pression* of the spirit leads to *depression*. I knew what a burden trying to fit into a mold that squelches your interests and your passions can be. I knew how it could stunt your growth and stifle your spirit.

At the Pennington Institute in Silver Spring, Maryland, we have provided holistic health services and counseling to hundreds of men and women like Sonya. People come to us with depression, digestive problems, insomnia, anxiety, and low self-esteem. We see people struggling with obesity and drug and substance abuse. We see women in menopause and victims of rape. We see chronic diseases such as hypertension, fibromyalgia, and more. The people who come to us are hungry for a different approach to wellness. They don't want prescriptions and pills and medicalese. They want a deeper understanding of what's troubling them. They don't want to focus on their bodies anymore: they want to move on to the business of *living*. They want to be healed on all levels.

This was not the approach that I saw in the medical establishment when I went into practice on my own. I had grown up watching my mother, Dr. Abigail Pennington, practice medicine at the hospital where she worked. I'd always seen her giving extra time and attention, caring for her patients' minds and spirits as well as their bodies. My mother went into medicine as a young woman to try to prevent anyone from dying as *her* mother had died. Her mother was obese and had hypertension but paid no attention to her health. She died when my mother was eleven years old. My mother practiced internal and geriatric medicine for many years. She was also an early user of acupuncture to successfully treat addiction to crack cocaine and other substances. Dr. P, as her patients call her, always believed in her patients' capacity to make evolutionary life changes. She has worked for more than twenty-five years now with people in every season and stage of life, serving not only as a physician and acupuncturist but as a counselor and healer as well. Quite apart from the physical treatment she might prescribe, my mother always took care to stress the *behavioral* choices that could offer her patients freedom from disease and mental anguish and enrich their lives. Patiently, she would guide them through relationship issues, stress, depression, and anxiety, helping them look deep inside themselves to find and remove the pebbles in the shoes of their subconscious mind, if you will, so they could live more fully and joyfully.

When I went into practice in pediatrics, I saw many of my colleagues focus on superficial issues and neglect some of the underlying psychological and emotional problems the family was facing. I felt that traditional medical practice was missing something. I thought, Wait a minute—that's not right! A doctor is supposed to be compassionate and really *dig* and help people get to the bottom of the issues that are troubling them. Over the last several years, my mother and I have joined forces to provide such an approach. The Pennington Institute is an integrative medicine facility: We are medical doctors, but we do acupuncture, psychological counseling, behavior modification, and stress management. We even have a therapeutic spa and salon within the facility, so that we can help people who are healing from bad relationships or getting over addictions to become more comfortable with their physical bodies.

Together, my mother and I have counseled hundreds of individuals, couples, and families, employing the principles we describe in this book. We instruct our patients how to tap into and channel the power of the mind, discipline and direct their bodies, and embrace and surrender to their spiritual calling. Many have undergone dramatic spiritual, physical, and emotional recoveries by applying this knowledge. Over time, Dr. P and I refined a set of simple life principles that can be applied to nearly any problem to produce improvement in health and well-being. Thus the Pennington Plan was created to provide guidance and help for our patients to reach their goals.

As distressed and depressed as our patients are, they come to us in an act of hope, and I saw a faint glimmer of that hope in Sonya's eyes that day. I suggested that in addition to treating her physical symptoms, we could work through some of her broader concerns by applying the Pennington Plan to her health and life situation. I explained that it would involve a very creative process, including a variety of homework assignments and exercises to help work through issues. Sonya was grateful to be able to explore and explain her feelings, and she knew that I understood where she was coming from. She saw no signs of judgment in my face, which made her feel comfortable and safe. Her eyes brightened with excitement. She wanted *permission* to explore new career ideas. I saw that somewhere inside she still held out hope—as so many of us do—of finding greater meaning in her life.

I began with Sonya by outlining the same concepts you will learn in this book. In the process, we agreed to tap into her spiritual desires by exploring some other career ideas that had been bubbling inside her for the last several years. She had dismissed these as silly fantasies, something she might pursue one day, in some distant future. On the contrary, I said: from my vantage point, the whole world was laid right here at her feet. The rules imposed by her parents, society, religion, and that misguided school counselor were not valid here, I explained. The only rule we would encourage and enforce was open exploration. "Ask yourself, 'What if I tried career X, or vocation Y?'" I said. "Ask yourself what it is you really want to do—and then do it." This may sound simplistic to some, but Sonya took it as permission to explore and indulge in all of the things that were tugging at her spirit. By asking a few simple questions of her true self,

Sonya found answers tumbling from the depths of her soul. What if I opened my own café? What if I started a women's help group?

All too often our true, inner self knows what it needs, if only we would take the time to really stop and listen. Imagine yourself driving a bus full of rambunctious children, trying to navigate rush-hour traffic and avoid the many potholes as the kids yell and scream. When you finally drop all of the children off, you pull to the side of the road to catch your breath, and you find that there is one child left sitting quietly in the back. You motion for her to come forward, and she comes to the front of the bus. "Where's your stop, dear?" you ask wearily, but instead of answering, she quietly begins to tell you of places she would like to see. Could you go and see them together, she wonders, now that the other kids are gone? You have to admit the sights she describes sound really inviting. But you're so tired. Who has time for this? you think. We need to get home and get some rest. Tomorrow we have to get up and do the whole route again. Don't we?

The child in the back of the bus is your true self. She wants your attention because she knows different ways of getting through town, with exciting sights and stops along the way. She wants to encourage you to try some alternate routes. But your true self is quiet and unassuming. If you allow louder voices to drown her out, you simply won't hear her. On the other hand, if you will just allow yourself to follow her guidance, you will discover that your true self really *does* know better ways to navigate these streets and new destinations that can become a source of joy. If you can quiet the mind and let your spirit express itself, you'll find that living with guidance from within can be far more rewarding than carrying the heavy burden of others' thoughts and opinions.

Sonya learned that this is what happens when we finally allow our spirit to spill forth with its true desires. She ultimately brought her artistic tendencies and caring nature together with the need to make a living by starting her own wardrobe and image-consulting business, and she has just completed classes to become a certified life coach. Sonya's physical complaints and insomnia have gone away as well. Her story demonstrates how intricately connected the mind, body, and spirit are. She learned that denying her spirit led to mental and physical manifestations, as the following diagram shows:

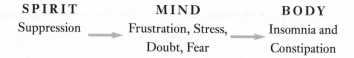

SPIRIT	MIND	BODY
Suppression	Frustration, Stress, Doubt, Fear	Insomnia and Constipation

I have known other patients like Sonya, who after years of denying abuse or internalizing stress or fear have been diagnosed with irritable bowel syndrome, infertility, uterine fibroids, and a host of other symptoms. Poor eating habits, lack of sleep, inactivity, smoking, excessive alcohol consumption—even a lifelong habit of unkindness or aggression—will sooner or later destroy the balance of the body and mind. Clinical studies have shown that consistent negative moods and thought patterns can depress your immune system, reducing your ability to fight infection and recover from illnesses or surgery. The functions of the digestive tract, reproductive organs, and heart and circulatory systems are all adversely affected by energy-dampening behaviors and thoughts. Your body simply cannot perform at its best when you live in an excess of negative emotion, internal turmoil, and dread. These feelings manifest themselves physically. Doubt, fear, anger, jealousy, and bitterness actually cause physical and biochemical imbalances in the body. Dis-ease leads to disease.

I do not suggest that illness does not affect the pure in heart and deed. But the *suffering* that often accompanies illness comes as a result of pessimism and self-destructive vices. Those with peace of mind, those who practice positive thinking, are often able to transcend their illnesses or attain their desires in spite of them. This concept is the cornerstone of numerous support groups; it has helped people overcome cancer and other, often fatal illnesses. The Pennington Plan makes use of this life-enhancing principle.

My mission is to help you discover and utilize once more your natural inner capacity for optimal health and emotional functioning. I have found that with sufficient desire, belief, and dedication, one can make almost any goal a reality. Desire, belief, and dedication are integral components of the Pennington Plan. I will teach you how to put them to use in your life right now. Once you balance and integrate your spirit, mind, and body, no physical illness will be able to stop you from living your destiny, and you will achieve the state of being known as wellness. What we are doing in this book, just as we did with Sonya, is designed to raise your consciousness and remind you of who you *really* are. You will learn to resist the negative tendencies that block the expression of your healthy nature and to express those that keep your vital life energy flowing.

Following the Pennington Plan provided Sonya with escape, relief, comfort, inspiration, and confidence. She is successfully utilizing the principles we describe here to take control of her thoughts and life. You, too, can leave depression, illness, and pain behind—for good.

AFFIRMATIONS

Wellness is my birthright.

Wellness is mine to reclaim.

*I will embrace my whole nature by
balancing mind, body, and spirit.*

*I will allow the voice of my spirit
to be heard and observed.*

*I will embark on my journey toward
wellness with an open heart and mind.*

*I will begin to observe the attitudes
I display—both negative and positive.*

2

The Spirit, Mind, and Body

CHAPTER 2

Spirit:
The Source of Wellness

W ho are you?

If you took this question at face value, you would probably start with your name. You might add your profession. You might also think it important to give your age, gender, nationality or ethnic background, and maybe your religion as well. But ask yourself the same question in a deeper and more searching way—Who am I, *really?*—and you start to wonder: Do those facts really capture all of me? Am I more than this person I see in the mirror? Why am I here? Is there more to my life than work, marriage, kids, death, and taxes? While these questions cannot be answered in clinical trials or laboratory experiments, our work with hundreds of patients has suggested some answers.

The False Self vs. the *Real You*

Your mind is a part of your whole being, but your mind alone is not "you." Your body is a physical manifestation of your whole being, but your body alone is not "you." There is an animating presence within you that is described as *spirit*. The spirit might be referred to as your "higher self"—an animating presence, a vital energy, that is the true essence of you. It is the *real you*.

Your physical self, including all the attributes such as your age, gender, profession, ethnicity, religion, etc., is like a mask. This is your ego, often referred to as your "lower self." The word *ego* does not simply imply one's penchant for high social standing, recognition, or praise. The ego is a construct of the mind. It is a façade, a social mask, but it is not the real you. The simple self is formed with the influences of society, family, peers, religion, and the mind's interpretation of life's experiences. Here's how.

Beginning in childhood we get a sense that we are separate from others. We look into the mirror and recognize the image as our own. We begin to compare our physical bodies and abilities with those that we see around us. In general, we learn to mistakenly identify our life, and sometimes our value, by our physical attributes, accomplishments, and/or failures. Over time, we begin to believe the judgments of family, friends, and the society in which we live about our bodies and talents. In the process we become self-conscious, worried about what others think and whether they will praise us, approve of us, or shame and reject us. All of these early perceptions affect our minds and shape our sense of self. Thus the ego, the simple self, is developed.

This simple self, with the influence of the mind, is only preoccupied with the survival of your flesh and the advancement of your personality. The primary objective of the lower self, the ego, is to use the mind to analyze situations and craft solutions to preserve its own existence. Based solely on the tangible here and now, the world of the ego is one of perceived vulnerability and isolation. Sadly, through the mind's mistaken belief in our isolated existence, the ego is filled with insecurity and fear, preoccupied with warding off potential threats, often rejecting and lashing out at people and circumstances from a position of "kill or be killed." But the lower self is a false self. And since the ego's obsessions are not even relevant to your true purpose in life, aligning with it can prevent you from living life to the fullest. To achieve that, you must align yourself instead with your true or higher self, your spirit.

Your Spirit—The Source of Wellness and Destiny

Your spirit is that part of you that gives meaning to life. It represents your personal destiny. The real you is unique, and your spirit accepts and embraces this uniqueness: it does not compare itself with others to determine its value, nor does it feel insecure. Your whole life long, no matter where you are or what you're doing, your spirit longs to express your own inborn interests and passions, to express that which is inherently *you*. A life that allows the fullest expression of your spirit is the most fulfilling life possible. Exploring, expressing, and realizing your true self is the purpose of life and an integral part of the experience of wellness.

Your spirit can steer you toward the attainment of your goals. It knows—that is, it *remembers*—the way to achieve them. Something about your spirit seems to be in direct communion with the very force of creation, tied to all knowledge and wisdom. The spirit is never wrong. You can trust its guidance.

Aligning with your spirit will infuse your personality and character with passion and enthusiasm. When your spiritual energy is harnessed and focused, you will become a magnet for the conditions you need to fulfill your desires. Favorable circumstances and people will migrate toward you. Good health and overall well-being will infuse your body and mind. Regular access to your spirit will recharge your batteries and boost your ability to recover from illness and injury faster. Just give it permission, and your spirit will help you soar to heights of supreme joy and vitality. Later, we will explore practices that will give you access to the renewing energy of your spirit and greatly enhance your health and mental well-being.

Mind and Body: Props for the Spirit

Shakespeare said, "All the world's a stage." In the stage play of your life, your spirit is the leading actor. Ideally, the body and mind serve as props (rather than getting in the way), but neither the mind nor the body can play the starring role. Rather, your spirit seeks to integrate your body and mind in order to achieve and perfect its purpose. Your spirit can use your mind to gain knowledge of this physical world, to accomplish wonderful tasks and create elaborate plans. It can use your body to move toward its spiritual goals. The mind and the body are necessary instruments; they are parts of the whole. But they do not in themselves *make* you whole. That is the task of your spirit. Your spirit completes you. Only the spirit can bring passion to your role in the world. Only your spirit can create authentic art and produce an inspiring expression of an eternal reality. But it cannot accomplish this single-handedly. Producing the play requires *all* of your being—spirit, mind, and body.

What delights the spirit is not the completed accomplishment itself but the joy it obtains through expression, exploration, and interaction with others. The experience of your own life lived to the fullest is the standing ovation for the spirit's performance. So do not confuse accomplishment with ultimate fulfillment. If victory and achievement alone were the objectives of life, we would not see such depression and despair among actors, artists, businesspeople, the rich and famous. Many seemingly successful people find reaching their destination anticlimactic. The joy is in the journey, not the destination. This is why you can truly enjoy life even in the face of disease. Many who live their lives with debilitating illnesses attest that once they put their anger, hurt feelings, and self-pity aside, they tapped into their spirit and began to really experience life. They learned that the spirit really doesn't mind that the body is not in perfect condition, so long as it is available—along with the mind—to further spirit's purpose. Many who have been diagnosed with chronic conditions, especially at very early ages, learn to come to terms with their illness and really dig into their life purpose and find meaning. They, too, will tell you that the journey, the exploration, and the expression of their internal passions to the best of their ability is what makes life worth living.

You may have heard how people or circumstances can "break your spirit." The fears, insecurity, and doubts that your mind imposes can certainly stand in the way of fully expressing your spirit's deepest desires. Negative thinking and verbal self-abuse can leave your ego wounded, wilted, and scarcely capable of expression—but not your spirit. The hurtful words or actions, intentional or otherwise, of people around you—lovers, employers, neighbors, and even family members—may threaten to deflect you from your spiritual course. They might feel jealous that they are not fully expressing their spiritual destiny and so may attempt—even subconsciously—to derail you. They may temporarily pull you off course, but they cannot truly silence your spirit. They may cause you to doubt its voice, but they can't break it. Even personal tragedy, loss, and sickness cannot break your spirit. The inspiring story of a woman who endured a tragic accident demonstrates this well.

Jessica's Story

Jessica was a thirty-five-year-old manager at a marketing firm, where she produced artwork and graphics for national advertising campaigns. She liked, but did not love, her job. Her true passion was oil painting, but using her artistic talents in marketing gave her financial security and stability. Jessica enjoyed a happy relationship with a man she loved and was in what she then considered to be the prime of her life when tragedy struck. Just after midnight, when Jessica was driving home from a coworker's housewarming party, a drunk driver crossed over the median on the roadway and hit her car head-on. Her airbag deployed and pinned her in the vehicle. Smoke from the engine billowed into the car's main compartment and she lost consciousness.

Badly burned and still unconscious, Jessica was eventually pulled from the wreckage. She was taken to a nearby trauma center where she underwent several operations. She woke up four days later, groggy and confused. Her memory of the events leading up to her hospitalization was fuzzy. At her bedside was her boyfriend, Eric, whom she recognized immediately. As her eyes fluttered open, he quickly went to her side and brushed away the tears falling down her cheeks. He smiled as she recognized his face and grabbed his hand. Eric leaned over the bed to hug Jessica. As she tried to scoot over toward him, she gasped in pain and horror. She raised her head and found that both of her legs had been amputated. The fire had burned her legs so badly that they could not be saved, even with skin grafting and multiple surgeries.

Jessica was devastated. She was furious at the senselessness of the accident that claimed her legs. Feeling robbed of her life, she fell into a profound depression, which severely hampered her rehabilitation process. She went through the strength-building exercises only half-heartedly. She did not want to speak to friends or family members and rejected her boyfriend's offers to work with her treatment team at the training center. Finally, she stopped going to her physical therapy sessions altogether. She shut herself in her apartment and shut out the rest of the world. She had no appetite, refused most meals that were offered to her, and began losing weight.

Months later, Eric, with the help of Jessica's sister, got her re-admitted to the hospital. This act saved her life. At first Jessica just sat listlessly looking out of the hospital window. She still would not engage in conversation with hospital staff, Eric, or her family, and she had to be nourished intravenously as she refused to eat. But as Jessica fell deeper and deeper into a state of helplessness and hope-lessness, something happened. She describes it today as her "light-bulb moment." For months, she said, her entire life seemed gray. She felt life had nothing more to offer her than a bleak, dull exis-tence. Many times she wished for death and begged God to take her away from it all.

Sitting in that hospital room, I felt like I was in a little dusky, gloomy box. Even my insides felt gray. Then, all of a sudden, I saw a dim light come on—*inside* of me. I know it sounds bizarre, but I literally "saw" a faint light flicker inside my heart. It was dim at first but gradually became brighter and brighter. It made me feel warm, and a rush of energy pulsed through me. I had never been a religious or particularly spiritual person, but I knew that this was something more than just a physical thing. My spirit came alive.

Gradually I felt a sense of calm, and peace, and relief. I won-dered if God was finally answering my prayer, and I wondered if

I was going to die. Warm tears streamed down my face, and I got a vision of myself painting. Just like my college days, I was painting with joy, listening to music, and singing as I rapturously engrossed myself in my work. The vision instilled within me such an intense joy and sense of purpose that I unconsciously called out. A nurse appeared in my doorway and was startled to find me red in the face, with tears streaming from my eyes. I asked her to bring me the art supplies that Eric brought weeks earlier in attempts to cheer me up, and I began to paint. I was not worried about whether I would be a "starving artist" or whether anyone would buy them. I just gave my soul what it asked for.

Jessica found that no matter the condition of her body, her true self simply wanted expression through oil painting. She realized that an inner strength that had always been with her was motivating her to look beyond her amputations to a new life. Though she described her life before the accident as meaningful and happy, she confesses that, in most ways, the accident was the best thing that happened to her. Through it, Jessica began living her destiny again. After her lightbulb moment, Jessica completed her rehabilitation with ease and emerged from her depression. She now uses prosthetic limbs to walk and describes herself as full of life. She is selling her paintings to hospitals and rehabilitation centers around the country. She and Eric have gotten engaged and are looking forward to their lives together.

Tragedy is but one way to tap into your inner drive for wellness. It may have been what led you to buy this book. But don't wait until you hit rock bottom: start seeking your inner source now. What beliefs, regrets, or actions are preventing you from living a fulfilled life? Your spirit may be able to provide the answers.

Becoming Aware of Your Spirit

The spirit, your source of wisdom, can reveal the origins of the pain, frustration, and doubt that have prevented you from being well and living your destiny. In many cases, you will discover the actions, beliefs, or fears that held you back from attempting and accomplishing your dreams or even led to physical illness. Your spirit knows the solutions to your questions or problems; they lie within. It makes them available to you without judgment. By simply asking your spirit for answers, you will discover how to recover wellness, learn what you *really* want from life, and explore ways to express your innermost desires.

Ask Questions of Your Spirit

Merely by posing the following questions to your spirit, you are declaring your intention to align with your true self and begin the healing process. You may not hear or receive all of the answers at this moment, but that is fine. The spirit never stops wanting to express its God-given destiny, and so the answers will come in time. Though you are asking questions with your mind, it will be the spirit that offers the truthful response to each. In time you will learn how to discern the difference between your mind/ego's automatic, analytic response and that of your true self. Just as you knew as a child that walking was something you wanted to master, you will naturally resonate with assurance when the right answers are presented to you. This may sound a bit nebulous for now, but it will become clearer. Just ask these questions, or come up with your own, and jot down any answers, sensations, or thoughts that are offered to you.

- *What is the source of my pain and discomfort?*

- *Which of my present attachments are holding me back from the experience of wellness?*

- *Am I holding on to past hurts with resentment, shame, or guilt? What are they?*

- *Have I allowed a fear of failure (or success) to render me hesitant, inactive, or stagnant?*

- *Have I allowed fear or doubt to stifle my passion and creativity?*

- *Am I judging myself against false or unrealistic standards?*

- *Are there people or situations that are preventing me from improving my well-being?*

- *What do I really want from life?*

- *How can I cultivate my sense of self and enjoy life again?*

Do not worry about what society, your church, parents, or partner think the answers *should* be. Let these questions filter into your deeper consciousness. Your spirit will hear them and will soon respond with such clarity that you will have no doubt about what may be keeping you from living a more rewarding life. As answers, feelings, messages, and thoughts come to you, do not analyze them. Do not judge them. Just take note of them and record them in your journal as you go along. Don't worry if only single words or incomplete phrases come to you. Write them down. They will become clearer as we go on.

Getting in touch with your true self will give you a glimpse of what life can be like when you are not trapped in your body or mind. You may feel a tingle of excitement as your true self impresses hints and suggestions upon you. You may sense a rush of healing current coursing throughout you. You may begin to receive inspiration and instruction to investigate a new treatment or intervention. Go with it! Your journey will bring you joy. Whatever the change, whether subtle or profound, you will begin to see how you can shift your focus to incorporate new activities, exploration, and fun into your life.

Get out of your mind and into your heart. Don't let your mind overanalyze your dreams and visions, and don't second-guess what is happening. Don't allow your mind to become an instrument of doubt and fear in service to the false self. Your mind is meant to serve the spirit, the real you, not the ego. In the realm of the spirit, there are no limitations. Only the mind imposes limitations. It doesn't matter whether you currently have the skills, resources, or physical capability to achieve your aspirations. And it really doesn't matter if your pursuits will take years to complete. Aligning with your spirit will bring you resources and contacts with the very situations and people that will help you achieve your dreams. The real you is never wrong. Even if you don't change careers or change relationships, staying in tune with your true self will make you more effective in everything you do, give your life new meaning, and turn even the simplest things into causes for celebration.

Using Your Mind as a Bridge to the Spirit

The mind can serve as a bridge to your spirit. Most people's minds are full of busy thoughts, noise, and confusion. This incessant racket prevents you from hearing, and thus responding to, your spirit's inner voice. To hear the soft and subtle voice of your true self you must first quiet your mind. Becoming still and quiet will open your mind up to ideas so illuminating that they are certain to improve your life.

Your spirit can in turn give your mind the insight and confidence it needs to re-create wellness and achieve your fondest dreams. As you begin to identify repressed emotions and confront the subconscious beliefs that have so far limited your success, your spirit can calm your troubled mind and prompt you to see things from a better perspective. It can guide and inspire you to more life-affirming beliefs and actions. By giving proper attention to your spirit, you will learn that you cannot fail. But you must make a *conscious* choice to tap into and follow the spirit's wisdom and direction.

You may not actually hear a voice per se as you begin this practice, so do not listen for one. The messages of the spirit often come as intuition, a sixth sense or gut feeling. You may sense a sudden urge or impulse to do something or to see someone. You may feel guided or led to action. You may receive a premonition or a hunch. Sooner or later, though, you will become conscious of something being said to you that you must act upon. Follow these impulses; they are seldom wrong.

Let's explore some ways you can lower the volume of your mind's internal chatter and hear the voice of your spirit.

Meditate

Meditation is the mental discipline of mindfulness, attentiveness, and awareness. In meditation you slow the flow of your thoughts by focusing your mind on a word, a mantra, or an activity, like deep breathing. Meditation produces a peaceful state that brings clarity to thought and access to the spirit.

Meditation can be a very helpful tool for tapping into your spiritual center and calming your senses. Oftentimes, during meditation, you will receive clear guiding impulses. Other times meditation will simply create the stillness your mind needs to access the spirit for an answer to a problem. You may find the answer delivered to you at a later time, usually when you're not thinking about the problem.

Meditation is good for your body as well. Studies have shown that meditation reduces anxiety. Meditation also helps to improve health by lowering blood pressure and decreasing the stress response. Long periods of stress flood our bodies with consistently elevated levels of stress hormones: these can damage many organs and affect our ability to think clearly. Meditating regularly can lighten your attitude and help you guard against overreacting to the irritation and agitation of everyday life. Meditation also helps your body recover from stressful situations such as surgery or infection. I find that daily meditation keeps me centered, balanced, and in tune with the rhythm of life. I highly recommend that you make meditation a regular part of your wellness practice.

Focus on your breathing.

Let go of thoughts.

Quiet your mind.

Experience your spiritual center.

Seek Stillness, Silence, and Solitude

Slightly different from meditation, aloneness is a necessary part of contacting the spirit. When you physically remove yourself from the fray of everyday life, you are able to silence your mind and tap into spiritual wisdom. It is best to go to a place in your home (or elsewhere if possible) where you can eliminate everything that produces sound and distraction (including children and pets!). Turn off the television, phones, computers, and pagers. Create a serene environment to help settle your mind. This seclusion will help you get in touch with your internal source of guidance. Take time alone, in silence, to connect with your true self and experience your inner wisdom. The more often you visit your special retreat, the more you will enjoy it. The less you go, the more you will avoid it.

Oftentimes we think that our answers are "out there." If only I could ask so and so, we think, this issue would be solved. I learned early on, however, that most of the answers to my problems were already in-

Be alone.
Be silent.
Be still.

Know your true self.

You are guided on the path
to wellness and fulfillment.

side of me. I simply had to quiet my mind and remove myself from the distracting opinions of others to see and hear them. Solutions to problems would then bubble up in my mind without effort. Even life-altering decisions could be made in these moments of clarity.

Commune with Nature

If you just can't sit still in meditation and you can't make alone time at home, try spending time in nature instead. Connecting with nature will allow you to tap into your spirit and begin a quiet journey into healing. Visiting the mountains, sitting in a quiet park, fishing, swimming, surfing, or hiking in the woods are wonderful ways to still the frantic flow of thoughts in your head and explore the inner workings of your heart. Without the clatter of the normal workaday world, you will recognize that your spirit, like nature, exists and flourishes effortlessly.

Enjoy the quietness of nature.

Be inspired by the tranquil beauty of your garden, a park, or the mountains.

Access the eternal source of life and wisdom in natural scenery.

Practice Yoga

The practice of yoga also helps to quiet and settle the mind. The word *yoga* means "to yoke" and implies a tying together of the body and spirit. Yoga's breathing exercises and stretches (asanas) have multiple benefits. They create a sense of clarity and focus. They help dispel stress and other harmful physical sensations. They align your physical body with your spirit. Those who make yoga a regular part of their lives enjoy improved strength, posture, and flexibility. They also benefit from the tranquil calm that permeates their mind. I find that yoga allows me to stay in touch with and control my body while clearing my mind. In particular, I enjoy listening to yoga chants to silence my mind before engaging in the stretches and poses. There are many wonderful CDs in bookstores and record stores that explore the yoga of sound.

Explore the poses and stretches of yoga.

Enjoy the yoga of sound through music or chanting.

Tie together mind, body, and spirit and experience harmony.

Each of these practices can bring you quietness and clarity of mind and access to spiritual tranquility. I view them as personal treats where I can enjoy private "me" time without guilt. By shutting down extraneous mental functions, you stop draining precious energy from the real stuff of life. By entering into a period of silence and stillness, you tap into your own personal generator. This will not only recharge your spiritual batteries but also will help you conserve and use energy more efficiently. Make a habit of visiting a quiet retreat, practicing yoga or meditation, and communing with nature. By doing so, your body will perform better and you'll have fewer power failures. You will enter into the wellness domain and experience life more fully. Don't forget to record any observations and insights in your journal.

AFFIRMATIONS

My true self is spirit.

*I am unique, and I have
a distinct purpose in life.*

*By accessing my spirit, I gain
awareness and understanding.*

I am guided from within.

*I trust my spirit for
strength and encouragement.*

*I will access my spirit regularly
for guidance and peace.*

*I will quiet my mind by retreating to a
private place, communing with nature,
meditating, practicing yoga, or chanting at
least two or three times each week.*

CHAPTER 3

Mind:
The Great Governor of Life

There are machines today that can take over the functions of your lungs, kidneys, and even your heart. But there is no artificial brain or mind that can sustain meaningful life for the body. In a sense, your mind is the most important part of you, since it controls all of your body's functions. But it does much more than that: whether your life is filled with health or infirmity, happiness or sadness, wealth or poverty is all determined in the mind. We humans have the unique ability to translate the images we create and hold in our minds into physical reality. Your mind's thoughts and moods prompt your behavior and determine your habits. Your mind cannot always dictate your experience, but it dictates the *quality* of your experience through the way it *perceives* that experience. Your mind determines your life achievements (and failures), articulating your goals, generating the ideas and motivation you use to accomplish them, and steering you along the way. Your imagination is so powerful that it can manifest your deepest desires and fears—whether abstract or concrete—on the physical plane. Much of this is accomplished with very little conscious thought. The mind is truly the master of the body: it has a profound impact on your health and well-being. Even conventional medicine now recognizes the mind's importance in our body's functioning—and malfunctioning.

One effect of this intricate connection between your mind and body is that the ideas you hold about illness and your vulnerability to infection can shape your body's reaction to stress and susceptibility to dis-ease. In fact, your subconscious beliefs can affect all of the body's organs, including those in the immune, respiratory, and cardiac systems. Buried hurts, resentment, and anger that smolder within the recesses of our minds can impair the physiology of our bodies. They slow down its cellular processes, hinder its vibrancy, and result in poor mental functioning and physical pain. Much has been studied and written about people who have suffered physical, emotional, or sexual abuse projecting their mental pain into physical discomfort and dis-ease. That which you think and believe, even subconsciously, affects your physical and mental health.

The mind's control over the body can be demonstrated with a simple example. Suppose you are unfortunate enough to be mugged. Your mind, in some almost invisible way, perceives danger and gives the alarm. The brain, which is tangible, responds with the release of chemical messengers; these in turn cause an instantaneous increase in heart rate and blood pressure as part of the fight-or-flight response. An entire cascade of hormones results in a series of physical and physiological responses designed to help you escape your attacker. In many cases, however, the actual assault need not actually happen: the mere *memory or thought* of being assaulted can trigger similar physical symptoms.

Conversely, the mind can induce a sense of calm and tranquility, even a decrease in blood pressure and heart rate, with the sight, sound, or thought of a peaceful setting, such as a beautiful sunset or calming music. Experts in mind over matter—that is, in extending their minds' control over their bodies—can apparently accomplish amazing physical feats of endurance. Firewalkers, for example, are able to walk on beds of hot coal without any burns to the soles of their feet. They consciously dampen the normal physical response to extreme heat so that, rather than getting scorched, they are left without a single burn. Others exert similar control over their bodies to withstand extremely cold temperatures. The Shao Lin monks, for example, can endure freezing mountain temperatures wrapped in cold, wet sheets for several hours and not suffer hypothermia. These are extreme cases, of course. The important point is that this same power of the mind is available to you for overcoming illness.

This power is a double-edged sword. The very same mental ability that can bring you good fortune can bring you bad fortune as well, according to how you use it. Just as you have the inborn power to improve your health and embrace wellness, you also have the power to create misery and perpetuate illness. You can, through focus and attention, intentionally channel the power of your mind to create good health and well-being. But you must be mindful of what you are doing, consciously focusing on life-affirming images and practices and shunning those thought patterns and behaviors that impose limitations and weaknesses.

With all of the elaborate functions that our minds control, wouldn't we be wise to be sure that they operate with the best of intentions and issue instructions for creating the most joyous, vibrant life experience? Let us delve further into the intricate workings of the human mind to better understand its influence and how we can modify and direct it.

How to Choose Wellness

Use the Mind's Paintbrush
to Determine the Color of Your Life

In every situation you find yourself in, your mind determines the quality of your experience—not the other way around. Your mind tints your view of reality with varied shades of judgment, mood, and outlook. This means you actually make a mental choice as to how you will perceive each encounter. For example, whether you see the glass as half empty or half full is determined in your mind. It's the same glass! Similarly, whether you regard illness as an impenetrable obstacle or as a challenge is determined in your mind. This is why the very same illness can knock one person into a lifelong depression and motivate another to reach for his or her dreams, no matter what. Your mind may color an encounter with an illness with shades of contempt, sadness, or despair:

"How worthless I am, to let a simple cold get me down like this."

"This is just going on and on. I can't imagine ever feeling well again."

"How sad and unfair that a person like me should be stricken this way!"

But you can also choose to meet that challenge to your health with optimism, grace, and courage, reinstating yourself in the realm of wellness by altering your perception.

Here's how. Imagine that, like a painter, you have many colors on your palette from which to choose when determining the overall hue of the painting that is your life. You may select colors like "bitterness" or "resentment," or you may select shades of "optimism" and "resilience." Circumstance does *not* automatically determine your experience any more than a painter's subject dictates color choice. You choose, whether consciously or not, how you color each of life's experiences. You have the power to color an encounter with illness with hues of "patience" and "hopefulness." Even in the face of a physical ailment, you truly have the choice to smile, to love, and to look for opportunities for growth and development. You can wallow in self-pity or look for the silver lining; it all involves intentional choice making. No one can make that choice for you. It is up to you to take responsibility for your thoughts and decide, once and for all, that you will look for every situation's brighter side.

Avoid Poor Little Old Me Syndrome (PLOMS)

Mary Ellen's Story

Mary Ellen was diagnosed with type II diabetes at the age of forty-two. This meant not only drastic and permanent changes in her diet but also a much increased risk of heart disease, poor circulation, and even blindness or amputations. While she was initially devastated by the diagnosis, she quickly decided that she would not allow her physical condition to rob her of her vibrant spirit. She was determined to live life to the fullest, no matter what. Her doctors told her that despite her diabetes, she could still control and maintain her health by following a nutritious diet and by exercising regularly. Mary Ellen grabbed hold of this advice and dedicated herself to keeping her body in top condition. Most important, Mary Ellen was unwavering in her refusal to succumb to depression. She knew that this, too, was in her power to control.

Mary Ellen had two sisters who died from very aggressive breast cancers. In the last years of their lives, Mary Ellen saw her sisters' vigor melt away along with their bodies. Despite their best efforts, the cancer and chemotherapy took much of their fighting power from them. Their emotions and passions, however, remained intact. Despite their physical pain and impending demise, Mary Ellen explained, they impressed her with their ability to find meaning in life. They each sought to reach out to others emotionally and spiritually. They told lively stories to their nieces and nephews, and before each sister passed away she asked the family about their dreams and aspirations. They offered love, blessings, and success to each family member with true eloquence. Mary Ellen said that her sisters had radiated a love and acceptance that was truly inspiring. She determined to do the same in her own way.

Her sisters' experience taught Mary Ellen that she did not have to allow diabetes to dictate her mood and disposition. She realized there was no use cursing her genetics, her fate, or God for her diabetes. She recognized that life often deals unfavorable hands, but it is up to us to play them wisely. Today Mary Ellen's life is centered on her passion, not around her illness. She feels that as long as she has the power to boost her physical condition and mental outlook, she will do so. By focusing the power of her mind she remains bright and lively and has effectively avoided the Poor Little Old Me Syndrome, aka PLOMS.

When I first met Ms. Jackson, on the other hand, she clearly suffered from PLOMS. Six months before our meeting she had slipped on a slick floor in the cafeteria of her workplace. Her fall resulted in excruciating back and leg pain, which kept her bedridden and on pain medication around the clock. She took a medical leave of absence, which led to inactivity, depression, and weight gain. She saw specialist after specialist, but each of her X rays showed her spine to be intact, and none of the multiple MRIs showed evidence of muscle damage or a pinched nerve that would account for her pain. She began to lash out at everyone. She fumed at the medical professionals who could not find a physical cause of her pain. She blamed her employer for creating an unsafe work environment and sued them to cover her loss of livelihood, suffering, and medical expenses.

Ms. Jackson came to the Pennington Institute at the urging of a friend, who recognized that her situation required a more holistic approach than X rays and MRIs. Normally home in bed with pain medication, she mustered up enough energy to visit us, leaning heavily on a cane. Our first visit made it clear that she was embracing and quite possibly worsening her condition to show that she was truly disabled and deserved financial compensation. I did believe that she was in intense physical pain; I also believed that it was perpetuated and made more severe by the profound depression and smoldering attitude of entitlement and bitterness that enveloped her. In the weeks that followed, her employer dropped her compensation to 50 percent, which only intensified her anger.

Addressing the physical manifestations is crucial in all such cases, of course. I began to treat her pain with acupuncture and therapeutic massage, which helped her decrease the amount of medication that she was taking. I also put her on a weight-loss program, using nutritional modification and supervised physical activity to help her shed the excess pounds she had picked up because of the injury. Dr. P. and I coupled this with psychological counseling and motivational support to treat her depression and anxiety.

We quickly discovered that Ms. Jackson had never really been happy at her job. She was an artist at heart, she said. Prior to moving to the area, she had designed elaborate ethnic art pieces, which gave her a tremendous sense of accomplishment and satisfaction—but didn't, as she said, "pay the bills and keep food on the table." So she took her current job, secretly blaming her employer for cutting her off from her destiny and never considering that she could pursue her artistic interests in her spare time. She allowed her mind, focused on visible circumstances, to limit her abilities.

But her mind, as Dr. P and I began to tell her, had unlimited power. We believed that with a change in outlook she could improve her mobility, lose weight, elevate her mood, and begin living her destiny again. She didn't buy it. "But I was wronged!" she complained. "The pain is real. They can't do this to me!" She went on and on reliving her trauma—all common signs of PLOMS. Your request for disability benefits may be justified, we told her, but right now you have talents and abilities that can—and indeed *must*—be expressed. An inspiring life purpose is critical to your good health and well-being. We explained that, anyway, her passion as an artist was not really dependent on her ability to walk without a cane. We said that by fully integrating and balancing her entire being—spirit, mind, and body—she could embrace wellness where she was at that moment.

After four weeks of counseling, including repeated affirmations and visualizations of a successful outcome, Ms. Jackson found that she *could* begin concentrating on the positive contributions she sought to make to the world through art. By that time she was not only walking without her cane, she was walking two miles per day. As she stopped identifying with her physical body and became less attached to her physical circumstance, she ascended from the depths of her depression and no longer suffered with back pain. Her energy and enthusiasm propelled her to a new plane of existence. She seemed like a newly liberated woman, talking and laughing and wearing more lively clothes. Most notably, she tapped into her spiritual passion and began creating art pieces again. Within weeks a curator from a local museum commissioned her to create several pieces for an upcoming exhibition. She had been cured of the PLOMS—and of her back and leg pain as well! Of course this did not mean that her problems were entirely over, but she had completely transformed the frame of mind with which she met the challenges of each new day.

Like Ms. Jackson, you may believe that illness is forced upon you by some external circumstance. However, when you recognize that *you have the power to create your experience* of each situation you face, you will discover that you can choose to deny the negative load and limitation of illness. It may seem difficult at first, but when you focus on the rich life still inside you, you will rise above circumstance, and your self-imposed restrictions will begin to drift away. Even if you are confronting a terminal illness, you can still seek to experience joy and exuberance rather than accept the depression and defeat that the mind usually offers. Illness may or may not be a choice, but taking steps toward wellness is.

Note the Influence of Your Subconscious Beliefs

Most of us, unfortunately, respond to an illness automatically and unconsciously. We react solely to physical circumstance and respond reflexively, based on the beliefs and assumptions stored deep in the vault of our mind—our subconscious. The mind fills in the blanks, if you will, applying its own brand of reason, one based on subconscious assumptions, to suggest a response to your present situation. But the mind is limited: it does not always perceive the whole story. When focused solely on sensory information from the physical world, your mind lacks a complete perception of reality. And our subconscious beliefs are too often neither life-enhancing nor wellness-supporting. On the other hand, once you realize that you may have imperfect programming at your core, you can replace it with programs of optimism, vitality, and health.

We discussed in Chapter 2 how the mind is involved with the creation and shaping of the ego. The mind incorrectly assumes that your physical existence is the ultimate reality and creates an identity based upon it. It processes information and feedback from your surroundings so as to shore up the perception of its separateness from others. The ego senses its own vulnerability and seeks to protect the human organism from harm and destruction, so it erects protective boundaries and initiates defensive reactions such as fear, competitiveness, and aggressiveness. These survival instincts become the very impulses that may prevent you from overcoming illness and living life to the fullest. But the ego, the lower self, is *not* the entire you. It is only a façade. Beyond the ego's perceptions is spirit, untouchable by physical circumstance and free from the threat of destruction.

Do Not Identify with Body or Mind

Ms. Jackson's case demonstrates that when we fail to look within, we're missing the most important piece of the puzzle. As long as we believe we are body and mind alone, we will be subject to the conditioned responses and reactions of the ego. Ms. Jackson felt unfairly put upon and helpless. She believed that someone outside of herself was responsible for the things happening to her, so she sought an external remedy for her condition. This belief was in the back of her mind at all times. When new challenges to her position arose, she reacted in the same way: she behaved as if she were being attacked and became defensive, angry, and resentful. Slowly, as she started to recognize and accept that she was more than flesh and more than mind, she began to recover. In particular, as Ms. Jackson reconnected with her spiritual destiny, she flourished. As instruments of the spirit, your mind and body require proper attention and use. But identifying *only* with them and neglecting your spirit robs your life of purpose and leads to disintegration of your whole being.

You become susceptible to Poor Little Old Me Syndrome when you identify solely with your body, illness, or pain. Like Ms. Jackson, you may feel limited, vulnerable, and defensive. But by changing your perspective, by recognizing that you are more than just your physical existence, you can change your life for the better. When you realize that you are more than flesh, as Ms. Jackson came to understand, you can begin to transcend the pain associated with it. Your existence goes beyond your physical body and its attributes. Your true self is spirit. By tapping into your spiritual power and channeling its energy through your mind, you can change your physical existence. You will need to examine your core beliefs and understand how they influence your emotional and physical well-being. If your assumptions about yourself are causing you emotional upset, physical unrest, or spiritual stagnation, they may need to be challenged and rewritten. We will expand on this further later in this chapter. For now, exploring the practices, such as meditation and yoga, suggested at the end of Chapter 2, will help you start to live from deep within, rather than merely responding to the outer world, and to manifest healing and vitality in your life.

To begin to embrace wellness, you must not identify with pain or illness—especially if your mind has colored your condition as dreadful. Remember, if you identify primarily with any one aspect of your body or physical history, that illness, past failure, or hardship will linger with you in the form of pain, dis-ease, and depression. Instead, like a child, you can begin to consider illness as only a minor wrinkle in the fabric of your life, rather than a fatally unraveling snag. For instance, do not say, "I am a diabetic." Instead say, "I have diabetes." Resist using your dis-ease to label yourself. Letting your physical manifestation define who you are makes getting beyond it much harder. Choose to see illness as one part of your life situation, not as your *entire* life.

Conditioning the Mind

So what determines how you will interpret your life events? What controls which colors you hold on your subconscious palette of perception? What governs the label or judgment you will stamp on your life experiences before storing them in your subconscious? The answer is conditioning. A lifetime's worth of impressions, beliefs, and attitudes have conditioned or trained you to react in certain ways and influence your every thought, mood, and behavior. Let's explore this idea in greater depth.

The Structure of the Mind

The primary parameters of the mind encompass the realms of memory, reason, and imagination. The mind stores past experiences as memories, applies reason to direct your behavior in the present, and through imagination conceives of your future. Throughout your life, you accumulate beliefs that are like reminders pasted on little cards and held in a storage chest in your subconscious mind: "Cold weather always makes me depressed and weary." "I always get sick with the change of seasons." These memory cards lie hidden just beneath the surface of your consciousness and shape your mind's reaction to the perceived environment. Unless consciously directed, the mind places the highest priority on your self-preservation. In this way, the conscious mind essentially acts as a pleasure/pain analysis instrument, relying upon—and creating—survival tips stored away in your subconscious.

All conscious organisms are endowed with such a survival instinct. The conscious mind appraises information from your five senses to determine whether a given situation will produce pain or pleasure. Those situations that produce pleasure will be remembered as potential survival enhancers; those that produce pain will be labeled as potential threats. The conscious mind has no memory of its own, per se: once it labels the object or circumstance, it files it in the storage chest of the subconscious mind. The mind thus behaves as a receiving, analyzing, and filing station:

CONSCIOUS MIND $\longrightarrow$ SUBCONSCIOUS MIND

Stimulus received and processed $\longrightarrow$ analyzed $\longrightarrow$ labeled $\longrightarrow$ filed into memory

The conscious mind compares each new experience to the memories of past experiences stored in the subconscious. It then applies reason to determine whether the current situation should be considered a threat to be avoided or a potential survival-enhancer to be embraced. Thus habitual patterns of pleasure-seeking and pain-avoidance are prompted by the subconscious mind.

Many learned behaviors come to seem automatic to us, but we *can* intervene; we can take conscious control over our mind to influence and possibly change its behavior. If you see a burning building, for instance, all your subconscious fire memories rear up to keep you a safe distance away. You could force yourself to plunge *into* such a building, on the other hand, to save someone trapped inside. With enough motivation, in other words, you could consciously choose to overcome the automatic response recommended by the subconscious. Such overriding of subconscious beliefs can be crucial to improving your health and well-being. You will learn to take advantage of this ability with this plan. The more you use it, the greater the wellness you will attain, on every level.

The Creation of Self-Concepts

In addition to "destruction-threatening" and "survival-assuring" labels of circumstances and objects, the subconscious mind also stores beliefs about you, your worth, your position in the world, and your abilities. Imagine that there are statements about you, your workplace, your role in your family, your country, and much more, all filed away in your subconscious: "I'm worthless, just like my father." "All the women in my family get fat when they hit forty." "Nice girls don't talk back to their men." The messages listed there shape the way you judge and interpret what happens to you, how you believe others perceive you, how you perceive others (including their motives and value), and what pursuits you consider useless or worthwhile. In short, they shape your entire relationship to the outside world.

Competitiveness vs. Creativity vs. Compassion

On the level of personality—beyond survival of your physical body—the mind will also judge circumstance and interpersonal exchanges on the basis of whether they will advance or hinder you socially. For instance, the mind compares your situation with that of others and will prompt an attitude of competitiveness, creativity, or compassion based on your accepted belief systems. A friend's accomplishment, for example, may make you feel jealous, proud and supportive, or indifferent. You may be inspired to reach for your dreams by seeing someone else do the same, or you may feel that it would be useless for you to attempt a similar project. It all depends on your points of reference, the self-concepts you hold in your subconscious.

The Influence of Subconscious Beliefs
on Your Current Condition

What you must come to realize is that any destructive beliefs or attitudes that were imprinted in your past may be affecting your health
and well-being now. They need to be examined and, if they are not
life-enhancing, changed. For instance, the subconscious belief that
you have less money than you need can make you very competitive
and aggressive when it comes to anything to do with money. You may
resent people with more money than you or those who seem to have
acquired their money too easily. You may be unkind to people whom
you suspect are getting favored treatment or who are competing for
the same financial rewards that you are pursuing. All these reactions
feed off the impression held in your subconscious.

When it comes to wellness, you may have cards stored in your
subconscious memory that warn you always to be on the watch for
threats to your health. You may go about your life in a defensive
mode, worried you'll pick up germs from bathrooms or airplanes or
someone else's sneeze. The opinions or experiences you gathered
about members of the opposite sex as a child may be shaping your
current attitudes about relationships. For instance, men who heard
that nice girls were quiet and docile may find that they secretly judge
and dislike women who are boisterous and outspoken—without even
having a clear idea why. Women who were told that life was about
finding a handsome man to marry, having babies, or attending ritzy
social functions often will pursue such a lifestyle without asking
themselves if it's really fulfilling for them. Of course these beliefs,
particularly if they are based in fantasy, often lead to disappointment. Some may settle for a situation that resembles their fantasy on
the outside but never fully make contact with that which is truly sat-
isfying. I am not saying that we cannot subscribe to any of the beliefs

our parents and society instilled in us; rather, that we must examine them to determine whether they are real to us as adults, particularly if these beliefs are detracting from our health and well-being.

For instance, we often hear patients in their fifties complain about their aging bodies. Their joints are on the verge of degeneration, they say; they expect their energy level to start plummeting any day now. They've just about given up travel or dancing: "At *our* age?" When asked, they explain that their parents or friends were just the same way. They accepted these examples as truth, a belief they have carried with them into their adult life. Then, as if a magical spell has been cast, they notice that their body indeed starts to "fall apart" when they hit the half-century mark.

Prophecies like these are self-fulfilling. People who believe that time or the world is against them will experience just that. Their subconscious mind prompts moods, thoughts, and behaviors that bring negative experiences in their wake. You've probably known someone who appears to have bad luck. Bad things just seem to happen to them more than good things. It's almost as though they have a dark cloud above their head, always raining misery. They catch a cold just because the season changes or because they see others catching colds. They project the negative attitudes encoded into their mind and thus attract negative experience.

Learned Helplessness

The idea that bad things can continually happen in a person's life because of what they are subconsciously projecting is not as unlikely as you might think. The story of Sarah illustrates this well.

Sarah's Story

Sarah was a thirty-five-year-old woman who was experiencing social anxiety and depression, which in turn was causing her to become withdrawn and lonely. Dr. P discovered that a string of abuses in childhood had led to certain thoughts and behaviors that may have reinforced the pattern of abuse and ultimately paralyzed Sarah with fear and guilt. Sarah's own words say it best:

> I was always smaller than other children my age. I was also quieter than any other kid I knew. Mostly because my mother always told me, "Children are to be seen, not heard." I never really spoke much or complained about anything because it was usually met with harsh words or a smack on the cheek. My small size and quiet nature usually led me to be picked on by other kids—in the family, at school, or by the baby-sitter, it didn't matter. If I told someone about it, they either didn't believe me or just wouldn't defend me. Dr. P says that's where I learned helplessness.
>
> When I was nine years old a relative sexually abused me and said that if I told anyone about it he would not only beat me up but he would continue to abuse me over and over. I tried to tell an older cousin but she said I was lying. I didn't tell anyone about the incident again until I was twenty-five, when I was seeing a therapist to deal with another sexual assault that happened in college. It wasn't until I started working with Dr. P that the pattern was revealed to me. Even now I'm not sure why I didn't see it sooner and put an end to it.
>
> In my current job working for a small accounting firm, another employer accused me of mishandling a client's account, which had resulted in an IRS audit and a stiff penalty. I began to wonder why so many bad things followed me through life. Is there a big sign on my forehead that reads "Easy Target"? Some-

thing about my inner beliefs and outward appearance and behavior was encouraging the world to take advantage of me—knowing that I would do nothing to defend myself. That is, until I learned that I *do* have the power to influence what happens to me.

Sarah's story demonstrates how beliefs held in the subconscious can influence our circumstances. As a child she had learned that when taunted or mistreated nothing she did mattered. Rather than learning ways to defend or protect herself, she had learned helplessness.

Over several months we began to help Sarah confront many long-held notions that she was weak, insignificant, and helpless. Helplessness, as Dr. P has taught for nearly thirty years, is not only something that some of us learn; it is something we can *un*learn as well. That is, we can change the way we think about ourselves and past situations using self-dialogues that create a much more rewarding life experience. Sarah learned to reevaluate her early life experiences from a different perspective—one that did not produce a permanent conception of herself as a helpless victim. She learned to recognize that, even though her family did not teach her that her complaints were valid, as an adult she was entitled to rewrite her self-description in much more liberating terms. She resisted for several weeks, but by gathering a mountain of evidence from her life since leaving home, she was able to be convinced that she has inherent value, and that her skills, interests, and talents make her a wonderful, worthwhile human being.

As we expose the negative imprints in our minds and become aware of their manipulation, we can consciously curb, and eventually erase, their influence. To free ourselves, we must move from unconscious, reactive behaviors to conscious choice making. The following story will help us explore this conditioning process further to learn how we can overturn it and reprogram our subconscious for good health and the experience of wellness.

Jonathan's Story

Jonathan was referred to the Institute for the treatment of a devastating alcohol addiction. Jonathan had hit rock bottom; he had recently been forced to give up his family business, nearly lost his home as well, and had narrowly missed losing his life in a car accident. He finally decided that he must put an end to his alcohol dependence. He was also being treated by a therapist for both obsessive-compulsive and anxiety disorders.

Jonathan was surprised that our intake interview included a detailed family and early childhood history. "No other doctor has asked such in-depth questions," he told us, "at least not about that far back in my life history." We explained that to get at the root cause of his addiction, we needed to better understand what experiences shaped his beliefs about love, family, money, and success. Understanding his points of reference would allow us to suggest solutions to his problems.

Indeed, Jonathan's intake interview revealed a great deal about the subconscious influences that were prompting his destructive behavior. His parents had worked nonstop, six or seven days a week, he told us. He and his older siblings were often left alone to care for themselves. They grew up completely isolated: they were not allowed to visit with other families or to play with neighborhood children and were told to stay at home at all times. The family never went on vacations together. Jonathan's father said frequently that money was the most important thing in life, and Jonathan's mother concurred.

Jonathan sought mind-numbing relief. He started smoking marijuana in high school and turned to alcohol in college. He was able to function well enough to achieve a C average, but he was usually treading a fine line between sober and stoned. During his college years Jonathan never faced the source of his emotional turmoil. Even at the age of forty-eight, he resisted any suggestion that he felt unloved and unappreciated by his parents; he simply sought relief in drugs and alcohol.

The painful experiences of Jonathan's early childhood left messages in his psyche that prompted him to pursue money over all else. The example his parents set by choosing long work hours over spending time with him and his siblings and emphasizing the importance of money led Jonathan to similar behaviors as a father and husband. Jonathan was obsessed with material wealth. He confessed that he felt no remorse for taking advantage of people in business, nor did he feel guilty for often neglecting his wife and child. He explained that he did not experience what he would consider normal emotions—happiness, affection, or compassion. He found himself incapable of feeling love or empathy for his new wife and their newborn baby. He was numb. He took joy neither in operating a lucrative business nor in having a supportive wife and healthy baby. He felt no positive emotions or comfort from his seemingly successful life. Instead, he once again sought temporary pleasure in drugs and alcohol. Only now, realizing that his alcohol addiction had almost cost him everything he'd worked for, did Jonathan feel an emotion. Now, he admitted, he felt terribly ashamed.

Together, we are working to help Jonathan realize that examining his thoughts and emotions moment by moment can free him to create the life he wants. Over the course of a few sessions, Jonathan's counseling showed how much he was suffering from what he felt was a lack of love, support, and interest from his family, and how much he needed relief from his mental anguish. He is gradually learning how the early programming of his subconscious mind continues to affect his thoughts and behaviors. For the past several months, Jonathan and his wife have come to sessions together. He has begun to go out on "dates" with his wife and daughter to relearn what pleasure feels like. His depressive symptoms have improved significantly, and he has been sober for three months.

Jonathan's story clearly shows us that the mind dictates what we do, when we do it, and how we do it. He has learned that the mind generates thoughts that we are frequently unconscious of, which in turn lead to feelings that motivate our actions. Jonathan's subconscious generated thoughts like "Mom and Dad chose work over me"; these led to feelings of worthlessness, which he attempted to drown with drugs and alcohol. "Money is the most important thing in life," his subconscious also told him, "more important even than family," and this led to his feeling aggressive and obsessed with pursuing material wealth above all else, no matter who was hurt in the process.

Thought $\longrightarrow$ Emotion (MOOD/FEELING) $\longrightarrow$ Motivation $\longrightarrow$ Action

These often flow from one to the next so quickly that we cannot see how we might interrupt the process. But we can. We do have the choice to slow down and unhook these elements and to choose the next step consciously. This is the first step toward reprogramming the subconscious mind and liberating you from the impulses and reactions that prevent you from living a healthful, robust life. The process requires focus and attention. It takes serious conviction that you want to change your life. But *you can do it*. This is what the gift of free will is all about!

What Is the Source of Your Feelings?

Highly trained neurosurgeons have cut open many a brain, but they have never seen a thought. Yet any one of us can consciously initiate thought at will or dismiss thoughts if we choose. As explained above, thoughts can produce moods and feelings, and these in turn can lead to actions. Because the process of thought begins in the mind, you can take conscious control over which thoughts will go on to produce feelings and moods and subsequent actions. In other words, you are not trapped by your past experiences or present emotions. Even if you have negative imprints on your psyche from childhood abuse or trauma, you can transcend and eliminate their influences. The chain that leads from thought to mood to feeling is in your control, whether you previously thought so or not. I remember how amazed one of our patients was to discover this.

Kevin's Story

Kevin was a forty-five-year-old man who came to see Dr. P for life coaching. His entire life was profoundly influenced by a delusional disorder, similar to paranoia, that had resulted from numerous subconscious fears of rejection. During his first interview, Kevin explained that despite being a skilled and experienced computer technician, he couldn't keep a job. He said that his frequent job transitions were always due to interpersonal differences beyond his control.

People always like him at first, Kevin explained. He has a lively personality and appears trustworthy: people tend to confide in him. His knack for solving computer problems quickly and effortlessly made him a great hire for any new company he encountered. But he seemed to bounce from one job to another and offered a different reason for each switch. One manager complained that he was rude to people calling for technical help. The complaint was false, Kevin said; the manager who lodged it was jealous of his skill and talent. He could not work for such a devious person, so he quit. In another company, Kevin believed that because he was gay, his coworkers deliberately kept information from him about special projects and excluded him from training events and classes. They talked about him behind his back, he said, and plotted to keep him from getting ahead. He finally blew up at them and walked off the job. Kevin recounted several other incidents with coworkers and casual acquaintances that allegedly mistreated or rejected him in one way or another. With some digging on our part, Kevin admitted that he had no concrete evidence in any of the situations to back up his claims of jealousy, sabotage, or secret hatred, but he just *knew* that people were against him.

We interviewed Kevin's younger half sister in an effort to understand the childhood experiences that led to his emotional turmoil. She had learned through Kevin's grandmother that their mother had been enjoying the carefree, single life of an eighteen-year-old when she discovered that she was pregnant. Rather than take responsibility for her actions, she blamed her new baby for the end of her freedom. She considered Kevin a liability, and it showed in the way she treated him. As a child he often heard her complaining to her friends and her own mother about what a burden and a nuisance he was, always needing food or attention. She treated him like an unwanted pest and never offered hugs, kisses, or praise.

Kevin grew up without the nurturing support of a mother figure and with constant rejection from his father. He recounted a sad story of how his mother tried to send him to his father's house for the summer when he was six years old. His father, having been similarly rejected by Kevin's mother for many years, decided to spite her by sending Kevin right back home. Kevin was devastated, and his mother offered no consolation. Instead, she accused him of ruining yet another summer for *her*.

These early experiences influenced Kevin's entire worldview. He carried in his subconscious the belief that everyone was a potential source of rejection. To compensate, he did everything he could to gain acceptance and approval: he studied hard and worked hard and was as kind and outgoing as possible. Kevin's half sister told us that everything he did seemed like the actions of a vulnerable little boy who desperately wanted acceptance and love—but then would sabotage relationships *himself* so as to avoid the pain of rejection. He rejected others before they could reject him. Once Kevin had won someone over with his outgoing, infectious personality, every encounter with them seemed to get shifted in his mind. He began to look suspiciously at every little thing that they did or did not say. With a bit more digging, Dr. P discovered that Kevin would rehearse scenarios in his head about how people were *probably* plotting against him and out to do him harm. He believed everyone was a potential source of pain and dismissal. He had a protective ego response of "kill or be killed." In fact, when probed, Kevin acknowledged that many of the people he preemptively rejected would call him to find out why he had left their lives—as if they were completely in the dark. "Kevin couldn't keep a friend if he paid them," his half sister said. "He needs help."

Kevin had a particularly hard time accepting the relationship between his childhood experiences and his adult behavior. It took him many months of counseling, visualizations, and a variety of exercises that you will learn in Part Three of this book, but he did slowly begin to form more normal relationships. Together, we had to consciously direct his thinking and install prompting cards of love and acceptance. To do that, he first had to face the dragons that lay in the chest of the subconscious mind. But he did it.

Are you ready to modify any negative beliefs you hold and improve your life? If so, you must first connect with your feelings to determine their source. What have you been conditioned to believe about the day-to-day experiences you face? You may need a lot of courage to address some painful repressed emotions, beliefs, or assumptions. But doing so can be absolutely liberating, for it will free you to focus on the life you want to create for yourself *now*. Again, this is an issue of conscious choice. You *can* focus the creative capacity of your mind to help you access the driving force of your spirit to break free from negative programming, defeat poor health, express your talents, and accomplish anything you want in life. Not everyone who had a troublesome childhood carries emotional baggage that haunts them as an adult. While I do not believe that everyone is hiding some terrible secret, most of us can probably identify hurtful events from the near or distant past that we keep experiencing.

Throughout this book you will learn many of the tricks we taught Kevin to prevent his mind from veering off course when his ego felt vulnerable. Take a few moments to examine your beliefs and write down your feelings and perceptions about the following questions in your journal.

- *What are my current beliefs about health and well-being?*

- *What beliefs about illness are stored in my subconscious mind?*

- *Can I identify the source of these beliefs?*

- *Was there a parent or family member whose opinions or behaviors shaped my beliefs about myself and how I should perform?*

- *Do my beliefs represent my current values and goals?*

- *Are they in line with who I really want to be?*

- *Do they really ring true for me now?*

- *Are there any beliefs about my health, my resilience, or my abilities that should be changed?*

- *What are my beliefs about my worth and value?*

- *How do these affect my relationships?*

Channel Your Energy and Thoughts for Good Health and Well-Being

All Things Come to Those Who Believe

How do you begin to enhance your physical health, mental functioning, and spiritual expression? By focusing your entire energy in the positive realm. You can consciously change and focus your physical charge by centering your mind on positive truths, engaging your body in regular activity, and tapping into your spirit. By accessing and projecting positive energy in the form of thought and action you will draw more uplifting energy toward you, and this will in turn make you stronger. Studies have shown that regularly thinking positive thoughts, smiling, and laughing can boost the immune system. In this way, positive energy may help to revitalize your body and mind and help you to achieve your goals. But your move toward healing goes beyond positive thinking. You must also believe that positive experience is available to you. You cannot simply repeat little affirmations and expect to see results if, at your core, you do not believe you are capable or worthy of health, love, belonging, and success.

Like calls to like. The ancient law of karma tells us: as you give, so shall you receive. The law of karma works both ways, and always according to your intention. If you exude negativity, not only will negativity remain but it will attract *more* negative experience into your life. When you exude positive energy, on the other hand, you will engage positive forces in your world that will help you rise above dis-ease of all kinds and realize excellent health. The same thinking and the same forces lie behind career advancement and good relationships. So beyond your thinking, you must become aware of the behavioral choices that you make every minute—until positivity becomes automatic. Focus your attention on bringing forth your own positive attributes to attract that which is meant to be yours—wellness, in all of its forms. Choose to *act* rather than *react*. Meditate on the positive aspects of life. Behave positively: by smiling and being kind, loving, forgiving, and supportive you will attract more positive experiences and emotions into your life. You will liberate yourself from the negative, limiting emotions that have kept you from feeling free and alive.

Remember, you *do* have good qualities and abilities. So get into the habit of disputing the negative ideas that your subconscious mind spits out. When you hear your inner voice telling you, "I'm no good at this" or "I'm always going to be fat" or "I've always been weak" or "I've never been as smart as . . ."—challenge those statements! You can say: "Wait a minute, now. Is this really true? Am I really being fair to myself? Do I really believe this?" You will surely find evidence to the contrary if you try.

The affirmations that follow each chapter of this book will help you to replace the reflexive thinking that your mind normally engages in. Let them motivate you to act in ways that produce harmony and healing. By memorizing and repeating them throughout the day, you will help them seep into your subconscious. To put this practice into place and let it start taking hold, I ask that you devote at least ten minutes each day in the morning and evening to meditation, sitting still, practicing yoga, or communing with nature (see Chapter 2). Ten minutes twice a day is all that I ask. First spend a few minutes letting your mind quiet down. Once your mind is still, repeat the affirmations slowly to yourself, or write your own to specifically address your desires for the day. In this way you will replace your mind's negative cue cards with positive ones. After a time, you may find that the benefits of just these ten-minute sessions each day will make you want even more. You will come to rest in the knowledge that you are not what your mind has led you to think. You are not alone in this world, but are connected to the source of healing. Your faith, also a positive force, will draw to you what you want and need.

As you stop allowing your mind to determine your behavior and mood based on what it sees in the world or holds in the subconscious, you will recognize that you have had an inner guide all along.

Naturally, if you spend twenty minutes a day affirming your rights to wellness and the other twenty-three hours and forty minutes denying them, you will continue to be troubled by limitation and sickness. So focus your thoughts on your positive affirmations throughout the day. Don't allow yourself to become a product of your physical circumstance; don't allow resistance or failure to convince you that the world is against you. Focusing on your limited mobility or pain will only bring you additional weakness and passivity. On the other hand, reject the tendency to perceive illness as oppressive, and you take a step away from negativity and toward positivity. Like calls to like. The negative energy of sickness can pull you down like a sinkhole. But if you choose to seek out and express positive emotion, thought, and action in the face of negativity, your positive energy will push back against those negative inclinations. The destructive, illness-promoting energy will soon depart. Your spirit has tremendous positive force. When you identify with your true self, your positive charge will simply drive negativity and pain away.

You have learned that your mind can be master or destroyer of your dreams: the choice is yours to make. You simply cannot allow your mind to impose false limitations upon you. It may judge the journey too difficult. It may cite past failures and offer reason upon reason why you cannot attain your goals or should not even attempt your new plans. Never allow this. You must channel the power of the mind to propel you ever closer to your destination. All circumstances can be changed for the good if you look for the opportunity. You are capable of producing whatever you hold most firm in your mind; so hold firm to your vision of victory.

I know that all of this is quite an undertaking, that I am asking you to replace the bad habits of a lifetime. As it takes time for better habits to take hold, I would like to suggest a way to jump-start the process. I have described in detail how negative thoughts and emotions can lead to physical pain and mental unrest. Now that you are learning new ways to overcome these negative tendencies, I want you to start exercising that conscious control. Here's what I want you to do.

Put yourself on a mental diet. For the next thirty days, I do not want you to think any negative thoughts. You cannot call yourself mean names in your head if you make a mistake or feel ill, and you cannot curse your condition in your head. If a negative thought should pop into your mind, replace it with a positive one. Dr. P often recounts the story of Elizabeth, a young woman whom she worked alongside for several years.

Elizabeth's Story

Elizabeth was a bright and positive woman. In the years that Dr. P worked in the office with her, she never heard an unkind word come from Elizabeth's mouth. She found something positive in every person and situation she encountered. She never contributed to negative talk. Quite the contrary: even when she came into the space of someone negative, she always had something positive to say. For instance, Dr. P overheard the following conversation near the drinking fountain one day. "Jones is such a jerk," one woman remarked. "He always has something nasty to say in the staff meeting. He can't even manage a compliment to his own team members. No wonder his wife left him."

"But doesn't he have the most beautiful smile?" Elizabeth replied. As she responded with kindness, Dr. P said you could almost see the other person jolt backward as if struck with an electrically positive charge by Elizabeth's kind words.

It can be quite dramatic how our energies, and thus moods and behaviors, can influence the energies of others. We always have the choice, in every encounter, to reach for the positive and allow it to lift us up.

Just as Elizabeth found something good to say about everyone, I want you to change the way you describe your life's challenges. Instead of saying "I can't do this or that," flip it and say, "I'm working on improving my ability to do this or that." Say things affirmatively; replace your usual negative rhetoric with positive affirmations. Become accountable for your attitude: realize that the attitude you bring to life is a matter of choice, not a given. Training yourself to align with positivity on the thirty-day mental diet will help you overcome a whole variety of health-related challenges that may come your way in the future.

Again, that which you think, you are. Whatever you focus your mind upon will be first imprinted on your subconscious and later brought to life in physical form. Focus on pain or limitation and that will become real in your life. Refuse to allow illness to rob you of your spiritual vitality, and you will spur on your body to fight off sickness and weakness. Yes, illness can come in without being deliberately invited, but whether or not it lingers or overtakes your life is determined by what you focus on in the plane of the mind. Make a conscious choice to view the illness as a minor speed bump, not as an impassable roadblock. You will then discover an increased sense of purpose and a remarkable drive to enjoy your life as the gift that it is.

Using the life you are given to the fullest can transform suffering into something sublime. We cannot determine the absolute length of our lives, but we *can* determine how we will use the time given to us. No one can promise us a tomorrow. But we can cherish and savor today, the present, as our gift from God. So look at life as a gift. Enjoy the challenge of the thirty-day mental diet and take notes in your journal as you make new discoveries!

AFFIRMATIONS

I make the circumstance;
the circumstance does not make me.

Illness may be a part of my life experience,
but it is not my whole experience.

I will flip any negative mood,
thought, or feeling around.

I will replace negative beliefs about
myself or my condition with positive
affirmations of wellness.

I will observe the attitudes I display and
look for the positive in all that I encounter.

CHAPTER 4

Body: Battered Warhorse
or Royal Chariot?

Our body can cause us great pain, largely because we do not properly understand its function. We have likened the body to a temple, adorned with jewels and sparkling paint. We have worshipped it like a deity. But most of the bodies we see in our medical practice are more like beasts of burden, battered warhorses. Their fragility has been entirely overlooked; they have been forced to carry loads too large for their frames and driven to exhaustion. They have been taken for granted, abused, ignored, and neglected. Some of our patients are so trapped in the pain or disability their bodies experience that they are unable to engage their minds and spirits in the flow of life.

The experience of wellness requires that we keep the role of our bodies in perspective. Your human body makes up only *one* part of your existence. It does not determine who you are and should not consume all of your focus. However, your body *is* vital to the fulfillment of your destiny. As such, it needs to be maintained and strengthened and given tender loving care. Certainly I do not want you to become obsessed with every detail of your body; I simply want you to understand its workings, the practices and rituals that will keep it healthy and how to limit the ill effects of dis-ease so that you can get on with the real stuff of life—exploration, experience, and mastery! Even if you are disabled or have a birth-associated deficiency, your body can offer you a lifetime of service for the achievement of your goals and the experience of many adventures—if you care for it properly. Each part of the body has a unique function, as this classic tale beautifully illustrates, and we must respect that.

The Rebellion of the Body

One day the hand decided that it would no longer deliver food to the mouth. "I do not hold this food for a very long time," it said. "I do not get any benefit from it, therefore I will no longer carry the food to you, mouth." The mouth replied, "I do not keep the food with me long either. After chewing it a while I swallow and it is gone. Therefore, I will no longer take part in this process either." Soon, the stomach joined the discussion and explained that it, too, would no longer deal with food, which, after all, passed only too quickly to the intestine.

On and on, each part of the body described how little it derived from the food and declared that it would no longer take part in its delivery to the next organ down the line. After all this discussion, can you guess what happened? Of course, the body perished. When each organ failed to do its part, the body could not survive.

So it is with your body. Each part must perform its function properly to ensure the survival of the entire organism. We've all heard the warnings from our health-care providers, the Surgeon General, and the media, but too few of us have taken the time to act on their advice or given much thought to the effects our daily actions have on our bodies. Is it possible that you are doing something that is harming one or many of your organs? Might you be depriving your brain, heart, or any other vital organ of the care it needs to provide you with a lifetime of proper function?

For instance, your heart is one of the most important muscles in your body, yet it is the organ we most take for granted. My proof of this claim is the sad fact that heart disease is the leading cause of death for men and women in the United States—and it is by and large controllable or preventable altogether. Surveys show that more women are worried about breast cancer and more men about prostate cancer than they are about heart disease, which is more common and claims almost 1 million American lives each year. Many of these lives could be spared with a little knowledge and by following simple health guidelines.

It is vital that we learn about the structure and function of our precious bodies, the ways they communicate illness or health, and how and why they can break down. Our bodies are complex and hardy machines, but ignoring their intricate details could lead to our premature departure from this life. Over the last several hundred years, ignorance of the mind-body-spirit connection and failure to engage our entire beings, as nature intended, have led to an explosion of physical and mental illnesses. Ironically, the conveniences of modern society have produced many contributing factors.

We move less. Technological advances have allowed us to become sedentary as we spend more time in front of televisions and computers. We don't have to search for, plant, or harvest our food. We communicate long-distance. We can travel long distances with no more effort than it takes to press our foot on the gas pedal. This sedentary lifestyle has led to more depression, obesity, high blood pressure, and heart disease.

We consume large quantities of processed food. Instead of whole food harvested from the earth, we often opt for highly processed products, microwave meals, and take-out dinners, many of which are stripped of their nutrient value in processing. Eating an over-processed diet can contribute to overweight, type 2 diabetes, heart disease, stroke, mental decline, high blood pressure, and even cancer. These conditions are prematurely robbing millions of children of their parents. They are largely preventable.

We stress more. We now live with constant stress. Decreased leisure time, consumerism, and increased commitments all contribute to it. Clinical studies have shown that prolonged exposure to stress hormones causes serious illness. Beyond ulcers and insomnia, chronic stress leads to heart disease, anxiety, depression, premature aging, mental decline, and perhaps cancer.

We are not mentally challenged. Unless we are driven to seek out new knowledge, we could easily spend all day just watching the images the media bombards us with. Many more people are absorbed in the latest sitcom than in any literary classic or new novel. This has resulted in dulled intelligence, embrace of mediocrity, and dependence on food, drugs, gambling, and sex for stimulation.

Gaining an understanding of the current diseases that are devastating our population and how to prevent them not only will help improve your physical health but will engage your intellect as well. In this book, I am not going to detail individual disorders and how you can prevent and treat them—there are many books, articles, and websites that can provide you with this information. I am simply putting you on the path to overall wellness, no matter what ailment you may need to overcome or what the mode of treatment may be.

In order to function at the highest level, it is critical that you obtain a thorough health evaluation to establish your present level of health and fitness and to determine whether you are at risk for one of these often-preventable health conditions. Ask your health-care provider for specific instructions on actions and activities that should be part of your personal health-maintenance regimen. Together you can investigate the treatments and preventive measures available to address any condition you face. Be sure to examine and discuss your family history. If you recognize a hereditary pattern for a particular health condition, use this knowledge to obtain regular health evaluations. If you don't already know them, at the very least you should know the following readings and levels that signal your risk for disease. Make an appointment today with your health-care provider to find out your:

- *Blood pressure*

- *Blood glucose*

- *Waist circumference*

- *Body mass index (BMI)*

- *Cholesterol profile (LDL, HDL, and triglycerides)*

As many of our patients discover, knowing these numbers can be the difference between life and death.

Keeping Stress to a Minimum

When we encounter stressful situations, our bodies release hormones that rev up our metabolic processes for fight or flight. The release of stress hormones such as adrenaline, cortisol, and others increases the strength of muscle contraction, raises our blood pressure, and heightens our awareness. In the short term, this is beneficial and preferential. For instance, if a robber were threatening to steal your car, the fight-or-flight response could provide you with the strength to fight him or the speed to run away from him instead. Once the threat or danger is passed, your stress hormone levels would return to normal.

Stress comes in many forms. We may only rarely be threatened with physical danger, but because most of our lives are filled with constant demands, we are constantly exposed to high levels of stress hormones. Your teenager comes home with *another* piercing. Work deadlines keep you at the office late for the third Friday evening in a row. Even the daily rush hour or the rise and fall of the NASDAQ can cause your heart to pound and your stomach to do flips. Unless you learn how to release your stress and quell the sometimes detrimental response, the hyperalert state produced by this elevated level of hormones can lead to serious long-term effects: nervousness and irritability, insomnia, ulcers, depression, anxiety, road rage, damage to your arteries, and increased risk of heart attacks and strokes.

How can something so vague and intangible as stress lead to physical damage of internal organs? Here are two case studies to help demonstrate and explain the connection.

Sean's Story

Sean is a forty-eight-year-old man who had suffered a stroke two months before visiting our office. His stroke could probably have been avoided. For three years Sean's body had been sending him warning signs, almost daily headaches that did not resolve with normal pain-relief medications or sleep. Sean had disregarded these warnings. Like most men, he neglected to see his doctor for yearly physicals, a simple checkup that could have diagnosed his high blood pressure and prevented his stroke. When he was finally diagnosed, his blood pressure was up to 175 over 100. Ideally, one's blood pressure should be *less than* 120 over 80. Sean learned that high blood pressure, or hypertension, is referred to as the "silent killer" because in the beginning, one has no pain or outward symptoms. Left un-treated, the pressure damages the heart and blood vessels and can lead to disaster—stroke, heart attack, or the onset of kidney disease.

Studies show that nearly one-third of all Americans have high blood pressure and don't even know it. Sean had no family history of hypertension. He was probably living with this silent killer for sev-eral years before it became obvious. Sean *was* aware enough to know that he lived under a lot of stress and was often angry and aggressive. What he didn't know was that such emotions and thought patterns so profoundly influence our physiology and body chemistry that they must be dealt with. Studies have been done to back this up. In 2003, the Coronary Artery Risk Development in Young Adults (CARDIA) study found that young adults with certain psychosocial factors were at a greater risk of developing high blood pressure and stroke later on. The high-risk factors include impatience, hostility, and "time ur-gency," the tendency to feel constantly rushed and pressured. If you, too, embody some of these typical Type A personality traits, you would do well to learn to manage them. The CARDIA study and many others constitute further evidence that mind and body are strongly connected and influence each other dramatically.

How high blood pressure leads to serious health consequences is relatively easy to understand. Our blood vessels are somewhat like rubber hoses. They bend, curl, stretch, and expand. If these vessels become narrow, then a greater driving force—higher pressure—must be used in order for blood to get through. When the interior space of our blood vessels is narrowed (by deposits of plaque, for in-stance, or by the thickening of the blood vessel walls in response to constant pressure), the heart must increase the force of its contrac-tions in order to propel blood throughout the body. The muscle thickening of the heart due to the increased pressure load is known as *hypertrophy*.

At first, the heart gets bigger and stronger, as any other hard-working muscle would, to handle the extra work. As in Sean's case, your heart can tolerate elevated blood pressure for quite some time, even years, without outward signs or symptoms. Sean's doctor could see with both an EKG and an ultrasound of the heart that his heart had gotten bigger to handle the high blood pressure. The scary fact is that the heart can only tolerate so much, and continued work against high pressure can eventually lead to its failure. Put simply, it starts to balloon out—like the cheeks of trumpet great Louis Armstrong—and to operate less and less efficiently.

Another consequence of high blood pressure is heart attacks. As it attempts to pump blood throughout the narrowed arteries of the body, sometimes the heart *itself* is starved for blood. When significantly narrowed, the coronary arteries don't deliver enough oxygen-rich blood to keep the heart muscle alive. As it becomes weak, it no longer functions properly, and it becomes difficult for you to endure vigorous exercise or activity without stopping to rest, catch your breath, or to recover from chest pain.

As high pressure continues, the walls of the arteries will get thicker and stiffer in order to withstand the pressure. Eventually, many of the smaller blood vessels in the body get so brittle and fragile that they can burst when the pressure rises further. This is precisely what happened to Sean. His stroke was caused by a ruptured blood vessel in the brain. The bleeding into Sean's brain tissue left him with limited use of his right leg. He is now receiving acupuncture treatments at the Institute to help in his stroke rehabilitation. He has completely modified his nutrition plan and takes medication to keep his blood pressure within the normal range. The same treatment, with regular exercise, could probably have prevented his stroke had he been evaluated by a health-care provider sooner.

By lowering your blood pressure (unless it is low already), you, too, can reduce the strain on the heart, which will allow it to return to its normal size and improve its function, providing it hasn't been severely damaged already. So please—do not neglect to get a physical exam and write down your blood pressure in your journal. Do not be afraid of the unknown. If you are diagnosed with high blood pressure, you can *beat* it!

Kent's Story

Kent was a fifty-five-year-old financial analyst who never learned to manage the stress in his life, with severe consequences for his health and well-being. For the last fifteen years he been driving his body to exhaustion, working long hours, abusing caffeine and nicotine, and eating whatever, whenever. He gulped down several cups of coffee to get himself going in the morning. He had a few drinks of alcohol at night to relax himself. Whenever he found himself depressed or unfocused, he would light a cigarette as a quick pick-me-up.

Kent soon found that he couldn't make it through his daily routine any other way. Even on the weekends, he found that his energy and mood were so low that he needed coffee and cigarettes to charge himself up and alcohol to come back down. He became edgy and easily frustrated, his irritability quickly turning into anger and hostility. He frequently yelled at his secretary, made unreasonable demands of his junior colleagues, and expressed extreme rage in traffic. He came to us on the verge of burnout: he felt totally out of control, he said, ready to explode at any moment.

Certainly not everyone has such severe reactions to prolonged stress. But studies have shown that the internal effects of burnout will catch up to you sooner or later. Our speedy, wired modern lives have many benefits. But we must begin to evaluate the costs, both physical and emotional, and develop a healthier course of action.

Chronic stress, nicotine, caffeine, and alcohol can deplete the brain of natural feel-good chemicals like dopamine and serotonin, leading to the types of reactions Kent was having. What Kent didn't know was that these substances can be replenished with certain nutritional supplements. You see, nicotine, caffeine, alcohol, and natural hormones like cortisol all produce a rapid release of neurotransmitters like dopamine and serotonin in the brain. Unfortunately, after continued exposure to these triggers, the brain can stop replenishing them in sufficient quantities. Having low dopamine and serotonin can lead to fatigue, low mood, low motivation, and irritability. The good news is that you can reverse these symptoms, with the help of your health-care provider, by cutting out stimulants like caffeine and nicotine and replenishing the neurotransmitters you have depleted. This was part of the solution we suggested for Kent. After a few weeks of supplementation, his body and mind began to function more normally. With the help of acupuncture, Kent established a regular sleep pattern and dispelled a lot of the negative energy that was brewing inside of him.

While restoring balance to Kent's physical state, Dr. P began working to bring harmony to his emotional condition. She explained to Kent that our thoughts often dictate our moods and profoundly affect the physiologic processes of the body. She taught him deep-breathing techniques to use during periods of stress to lower his blood pressure, calm his nerves, and distract him from angry thoughts and impulses. Dr. P also suggested ways that Kent might work consciously to change his reactions to frustration, particularly his road rage. Next time someone darts in front of you on the freeway, she told him, imagine that she is a dear friend who was a bit preoccupied and missed her exit. If he saw her as a friend, he would of course recognize that her zooming in front of him was not an intentionally reckless maneuver. Instead of responding with cursing or threats of abuse, he might be more inclined to feel concern for her and wish her well on her journey.

Kent fought this for a while. Those "idiots" on the road were no friends of his, he said, and they richly deserved his anger and name-calling. He was, at first, completely missing the point: his behavior was not even affecting the other drivers, let alone getting them to stop cutting him off. But it *was* damaging his own mind and body and could potentially put him in danger of retaliation or a heart attack. Dr. P persisted with her usual patience. If you can't imagine the other drivers as your friends, she told him, try seeing them as young, innocent children—anything that will help you treat them with more tolerance and patience. Compassion is a tough lesson to learn, but with a bit of counseling, it stuck for him.

What is the lesson here? That getting harmful emotions in check can be crucial to protecting your health. The mind and body are so intricately connected that your ultimate health and well-being depend upon your taking control of *all* of your being. The stress-management techniques described in Chapter 2—communing with nature, focused relaxation, meditation, and exercise—will help you maintain a youthful, resilient body, a sharp mind, and a calm spirit if you practice them regularly. You will find, as Kent did, that these can help release some of your tension and dispel the toxicity of the stress response. Also be sure to stick with your thirty-day mental diet as you retrain your mind to create positive, health-affirming thought patterns. Research shows that by adopting such belief systems you'll not only live longer—you'll also live better.

Rest and Relaxation

Our hectic lifestyles and the relentless pressures upon us leave little time for rest and relaxation. But studies show that when we neglect to give the body sufficient time to rejuvenate itself, we hasten the aging process. Lack of sleep leads to mental decline, irritability, and poor response to stress. Kent thought it strange when we told him to take ten to twenty minutes out of his busy day for a time-out. But taking a bit of "me" time will realign your body, mind, and spirit and allow you to function better. My typical Type A, overachiever patients actually find that they get better work done in less time when they give their body and spirit time to recuperate from the constant deadlines, incessant worry, and self-imposed demands. So, sneak away to a quiet room, or even your car, for a dose of solitude. Take five deep breaths and feel the connection with your inner source of peace and serenity. When we are busy and stressed, we tend to breathe shallow, quick breaths, which can lead to the retention of carbon dioxide in our lungs. Taking slow deep breaths will help you get rid of the excess carbon dioxide and will nourish your brain and other tissues with oxygen.

Also be sure to get a minimum of seven to nine hours of sleep each night—or, if that is impossible, to at least take a short nap during the day. Studies show that as we age our sleep requirements increase. The body needs time off from the high levels of stress hormones and physical demands of the day to recuperate, repair, and renew. Be sure to create a bedroom that welcomes rest and sleep. When we queried Kent about his sleeping quarters, we discovered that he had books and stacks of paper from work on his bedside tables. His television was aimed at the bed and provided background noise that he used to fall asleep at night. We told him that limiting the books and other clutter at his bedside and turning off his TV would help quiet his mind and soften his senses. We urged him to use his bedroom for rest and intimacy—not for work. Follow this advice and your body will thank you with years of proper functioning.

Proper Nutrition

Studies show that simply fueling your body with the necessary nutrients will help to keep all of its parts working optimally. A well-balanced diet will improve the look and function of your body and all of its precious organs. You can prevent heart disease, diabetes, and even cancer by eating for life, rather than only for comfort. Even your skin can look more radiant and supple and defy the usual effects of time if you eat right and drink plenty of water. The body only needs enough fuel to meet its daily energetic requirements; any excess will be stored as fat. Ideally, you should provide your body with a steady influx of just enough energy to meet your daily activity needs. Eating any more not only adds unsightly fat to your hips and cholesterol deposits to your arteries; it also makes you more sluggish. A good rule of thumb is to meet your daily calorie requirements with about 30 to 40 percent complex carbohydrates, less than 30 percent from good fats, and about 30 to 40 percent from protein. Talk to your health-care provider to determine the best ratios for your condition and lifestyle.

The following dietary guidelines can help you stay energized, provide the nutrients you need for healthy mental functioning, preserve your eyesight, prevent cholesterol buildup, lower blood pressure, bring a glow to your skin, and maintain a healthy weight—all without being starved or feeling deprived. It's easier than you think. By incorporating a few simple changes into your life, you'll lose excess pounds (if you need to) and may lower your risk for heart disease, diabetes, colon cancer, and more.

You should eat five or six small meals and snacks each day, every three to four hours. Do not eat past 7 p.m., or within four hours of bedtime, and try to avoid simple-sugar snacks such as cookies, candy, juice, and sodas. And, fads aside, a low-carb diet can be very helpful in maintaining a healthy weight. Get more fruits and vegetables in your diet by having a salad with lunch and dinner—full of fresh tomatoes, snap peas, cucumbers, bell peppers, carrots, and sprouts. Keep fresh fruit instead of cookies or crackers near your desk at work or by the front door to eat as a snack when you're on the go. And for that afternoon slump, instead of hitting up the vending machine, carry some fresh fruit or veggies with you to dip into some hummus or peanut butter, which are both great sources of protein. Personally, I love cucumber slices and hummus. Each time you eat fruits or vegetables, remember that you are doing your whole body a favor. They are loaded with antioxidant vitamins and phytochemicals that fight disease. These crunchy snacks also send a message to your brain that you are following its instruction to eat and your brain will turn off the feeding frenzy. For an after-dinner treat, try fresh strawberries or melon instead of cakes or candy. Or make a creamy yogurt smoothie with fresh fruits for a naturally sweet, refreshing way to increase your daily intake of fruits. (Diabetics should be sure to monitor their blood sugar levels because fruit can easily raise glucose levels.) You can still enjoy your favorite treats from time to time, but the key is to do so in moderation. "The sin is not in the doing," as Dr. P always says. "It's in the overdoing!"

Many adults have healthy eating habits but relax their vigilance with their children, who can be strong-willed and picky and are seemingly indestructible. The following story demonstrates how important healthy eating is for children as well.

Matthew's Story

Type 2 diabetes is at an all-time high among American adults. Among American youth it is an emerging epidemic. This condition was once referred to as adult onset diabetes: twenty years ago, only 2 percent of new cases were among children. Today, nearly 20 percent of those diagnosed with type 2 diabetes are children ages nine to nineteen. Type 2 diabetes can lead to serious complications, including blindness, limb amputation, kidney failure, and heart disease. Research shows that the main culprits in this growing epidemic among youth are alarming rates of obesity and a sedentary lifestyle. With nearly one-third of American youth overweight, it's no wonder this epidemic is spreading.

Matthew is a seventeen-year-old boy who, at a height of five foot three, weighed 195 pounds, putting him in the obese category. After complaining of fatigue, extreme thirst, and frequent urination, he was diagnosed with type 2 diabetes, and his physician referred him and his mother to the Institute for diabetes education classes. In his first session he told us he was afraid of being forced to give himself insulin shots every day. I explained that unlike people with type 1 diabetes, whose bodies stop producing insulin, people with type 2 diabetes still produce plenty of insulin but the tissues of their body don't respond to it. I also explained to Matthew and his mother that insulin resistance is seen in people with low physical activity and high body fat levels. I said that he could most likely avoid daily injections if he lost weight, exercised regularly, and ate nutritious, well-balanced meals. Matthew's lingering fear of shots gave him a serious incentive to lose weight, which was encouraging, since motivation is crucial in making and maintaining these life changes.

Matthew's mother was upset to learn that her son's condition could have been prevented. She felt that his diabetes was her fault. She admitted that because she felt that their neighborhood wasn't very safe, Matthew watched TV and played on their home computer instead of riding bikes and playing outside. His mother explained that it was so hard to get him to eat vegetables and other healthy dishes that she had given up cooking them. He was always begging for fast food and sugary treats. She blamed this partly on the school he attended, which served such things regularly. I understood all too well how hard it is to ensure that your children are eating well-balanced meals. Junk food is plentiful and readily available, including at school, as many schools offer hamburgers, pizza, and other high-fat, processed foods over healthier choices. At home, the busy American lifestyle often prevents families from eating healthful meals together, which keeps children from learning about healthy food choices, nutrition, and self-control at an early age.

I explained that to retrain Matthew to eat healthy foods and to teach him about the proper care of his body, the behaviors would have to start at home. I encouraged Matthew's mom to become more active physically to set a good example for him and his younger sister. I suggested that she begin by getting regular physical activity *with* her children and eating balanced meals with them as well. Because so many of our behaviors serve as models for our children, this type of influence can last for life. Matthew was excited to learn that he could improve his health by the choices he makes every day. I hope that you will feel some of the same enthusiasm on your journey toward wellness.

Physical Activity and Exercise

"Move it or lose it" is a crucial guideline for optimal well-being. Our bodies are meant to move. Inactivity weakens muscles, stiffens joints, and increases accumulation of body fat, all of which can increase our fragility and decrease our agility. If you were to leave your car in the garage for several months, it might run poorly or might not even start when you wanted to drive it again. The same holds true for your body. Getting regular physical activity keeps your heart strong enough to pump blood through the body, your lungs conditioned to provide vital oxygen to your tissues, your joints limber, bones strong, and muscles loose enough to move you nimbly throughout life. Your body will also be better able to use nutrients for fuel rather than storing them as fat. Playing with your children outdoors, taking the stairs at work, parking farther away from the grocery store or mall, and taking walks or going to the gym on your lunch break will greatly improve your overall health. Your health-care provider can help you create a plan for integrating exercise into your daily routine.

Exercise helps stave off depression and anxiety. It's true. You actually get a dose of natural feel-good chemicals, known as endorphins—natural antidepressants that are released by the brain—from engaging in regular physical activity. Exercise helps you achieve better blood sugar control, lower blood pressure, and lower cholesterol. Getting just thirty minutes of exercise on most days of the week can also help prevent many of the outward signs of aging. You don't even have to get all thirty minutes at once. Ten minutes here and twenty minutes there can add up to provide health benefits as well. So go for a brisk walk. Go bowling. Go swimming or dancing. Just be sure to get your body moving to keep yourself well and elevate your mood. Focus on your motivating factors as you do it, to keep your enthusiasm high. No excuses! No matter how busy you are, you *must* make time for regular exercise. Most people have heard that regular physical activity will actually help them prevent heart disease, diabetes, even cancer. But they still don't do it! Don't be one of them. Get moving!

Even if you have never exercised regularly in your life, it is never too late to start. As Belinda's story shows, with enough motivation *you can do it*.

Belinda's Story

Belinda is a thirty-three-year-old woman who noticed that her afternoon walks with her twins were becoming more and more difficult to complete. Her six-year-old twin sons enjoy rollerblading and riding bikes, and she began walking around the neighborhood alongside the boys to get more exercise and lose weight. To her surprise, she found she sometimes had to stop to catch her breath after just a few blocks. Though she was only thirty pounds overweight (or so she thought), she was surprised to feel so winded as she hit the half-mile mark of her route. Belinda had recently quit smoking and thought that having smoked cigarettes for the last ten years probably damaged her lungs. She had no idea that the cigarettes had damaged her blood vessels and that her breathlessness was a notice from her heart that it was starving for blood.

Your heart will beat nearly 275 *billion* times in your lifetime, pumping precious blood to every organ and tissue in your body. Though it is in contact with blood at all times, it requires its own supply to keep it ticking. In fact, the heart has its own personal network of blood vessels, the coronary arteries, which dive deep into the heart muscle to nourish it. If these arteries become blocked or narrowed, part or all of the heart muscle may be starved.

Belinda got more hints. She woke up at four o'clock one morning with feelings of nausea and anxiety. She thought perhaps it was a touch of worry about an upcoming visit from her in-laws. But after breakfast later that morning, she felt dizzy and more nauseated. One of her boys was getting over a bad cold; she thought perhaps she had picked up whatever germ he had and dismissed the symptoms. Not quite a week later, Belinda was walking with her sons to the local park when she felt an achy pain in the middle of her back. She felt sweaty and sort of nervous and apprehensive and called her doctor seeking reassurance that it wasn't something serious. He told her to come in just to be sure. What happened next is what shocked Belinda.

Her family physician suggested that, given her symptoms, Belinda should have an EKG. He also explained that with a body mass index (a number that relates your height to your weight) of thirty-one, Belinda was obese, which increased her risk of developing heart disease. Belinda was shocked. "Aren't I too young for a heart attack?" she asked. Her doctor explained that heart disease can strike at any age—particularly in a person with a family history of the disease. Belinda's mother, he reminded her, had died of a heart attack at the age of forty-seven.

Belinda couldn't remember what symptoms her mother had before the heart attack that claimed her life, but she was sure her mom did not complain of chest pain. Women often have different symptoms than men, her doctor explained. While men commonly experience crushing chest pain that may radiate to the left arm or jaw, for women the symptoms often include anxiety, nausea, dizziness, and fatigue. Sometimes the chest pain is minor and is dismissed as mere heartburn.

Belinda's EKG showed evidence of an old heart attack: part of her heart tissue had died due to decreased blood supply. As the doctor evaluated her further, he found that her cholesterol was 235 mg/dL, well above the recommended maximum of 200. Belinda's family genetics, cholesterol level, sedentary lifestyle, and smoking history made for a dangerous combination, her doctor explained, because smoking damages the blood vessels and makes them more likely to accumulate fatty cholesterol deposits and other cellular material. These deposits block the flow of blood and greatly increase the risk of heart attack or stroke.

Belinda was referred to the Institute for help in repairing some of the damage and to create a plan for health maintenance. She had unknowingly been damaging her body for years. She did not know that her family history put her at risk for developing heart disease. She was unaware that she might prevent this by exercising regularly, eating properly, and abstaining from toxic substances like cigarettes. Fortunately, atherosclerosis is reversible in many cases. We taught her that good nutrition, increased physical activity, and a positive outlook could help her to improve her health, clean up her arteries, and lower her risk of a fatal heart attack. Belinda remembered how devastating it had been to lose her own mother when she was just sixteen years old. She felt that she owed it to her sons to do all she could to be around for them. That gave her all the motivation she needed.

Belinda began a program of walking around the neighborhood and bike riding, nutrition counseling, acupuncture, and meditation. Her body, in turn, started sending her grateful messages of relief. She noticed that with each five pounds she lost, she had more energy. A tremendous sense of joy bubbled within her. Overall, she lost forty-five pounds and felt such a relief that at times she just wanted to sing—and often did, in keeping with Step 5 of the Pennington Plan. Belinda's whole perspective on life changed. Knowing more about her body, she began to treat it as a royal chariot. She learned and practiced good stress-management techniques. She gave herself mini time-outs to pamper herself and nurture her spirit. She started teaching her sons about healthy nutrition and the power of the mind and saw their creativity and zest for life soar as well. She began to view the warning signs she had received as God's way of telling her to treat life as a gift and to pass on this newfound knowledge to her sons.

Your own body, like Belinda's, is constantly communicating its needs, deficiencies, likes, and dislikes. If a little indicator light came on in your automobile you would either consult a repair shop or your owner's manual for guidance. In the same manner, if you sense something in your body that feels uncomfortable, ask a health-care professional for an explanation. Your very life may depend upon it.

But don't wait for life-threatening symptoms—start *now*, before you get sick. Don't stay in the trap of inertia and inactivity. Even if you can only squeeze in ten minutes here or there with a walk around the block, a small amount is better than none at all. Remember, it all adds up! But, as you have time, add longer workouts into your regimen. Ultimately, exercising will become as natural to you as sleeping in on the weekends. Remembering that you're actively taking steps to maintain your youth and health will give you enthusiasm and motivation as well. Exercise stops being a chore when you focus on the outcome. Instead, you'll regard it as an essential component of your self-preservation regimen.

Here are some ways to get your body moving. Remember: *Before beginning any new fitness regimen, please consult your physician.*

Exercise for strength. To maintain an upright posture and the ability to perform daily tasks (that is, lifting groceries or grandkids) with less likelihood of injury or falls, exercising for strength should be your goal. So-called "resistance training" is a wonderful way to improve and maintain muscle strength and increase bone density. By lifting weights or performing exercises against your own body weight, you may decrease your risk of bone fractures due to osteoporosis and stooped posture. Visit our website for simple exercises that you can perform at home.

Exercise for flexibility. To preserve your smooth step, include exercises that involve stretching, such as yoga or Pilates. Joint flexibility tends to decrease with age due to a decrease in the production of the fluid that cushions our joints. With decreased use, your tendons can become stiff and resistant, so it is critical to perform stretching exercises to maintain your flexibility. Not only will your ability to dance, run, and bowl be maintained, you will also be less likely to suffer an injury due to a fall or sprain.

Exercise for endurance. To continue to walk around the block without huffing and puffing, include aerobic exercise in your routine. Aerobic exercise conditions your cardiovascular system: it helps your heart beat more efficiently and your lungs provide you with fresh oxygen to meet the demands of an active lifestyle. Walking creates energy and stamina. So if you never had much energy before, start walking, and you will.

Nutritional Supplements

Once you have gotten your general health under control, your interest and attention may shift toward protecting your health investment. Perhaps you are facing midlife and want to prevent the onset of age-related dis-ease, for example. Clinical studies are showing that taking nutritional supplements to provide vitamins, minerals, and antioxidants can keep the body functioning properly and can be particularly helpful in preventing many chronic diseases and conditions associated with advanced age. Other studies offer strong evidence that taking certain amino acids as oral supplements can be useful in the treatment of mood disorders, like depression and anxiety, and can also benefit those who are addicted to or detoxing from alcohol, stimulants, like caffeine and cocaine, and prescription drugs, like benzodiazepines. Also, as you learned from Kent's story, amino acid supplementation can help aid recovery from stress- and drug-induced burnout.

Even in a seemingly nutritious diet, our food's vitamins, minerals, and important trace elements can be decreased by year-round farming techniques, food processing, and food preparation. For this reason I recommend that you speak with your health-care provider about whether you should add nutritional supplements to your health plan and ask for recommendations of the brands he or she trusts most.

The role of antioxidants in combating the effects of aging is worth expanding upon. Normally the DNA in our cells determines when and how our cells age and die. To a large extent, the programmed time of cell death is out of our immediate control. But one aspect of aging that we can influence is *premature aging*. Most of the physical signs of aging, such as wrinkles, stooped posture, stiff and achy joints, and poor vision, are brought on *prematurely* by environmental factors and bad lifestyle choices. Unless genetically programmed to do so, many of the cells of your body are not intended to degenerate until very late in life—if at all. Excessive alcohol consumption, cigarette smoking, pessimism, anger, impatience, pollution, excessive exposure to sunlight, inactivity, prolonged exposure to stressful situations, and poor nutrition all lead to cellular damage that accelerates the aging process. The free radical theory of aging, first introduced in 1954, explains how.

Normal cellular function results in the formation of highly reactive, terribly destructive particles known as free radicals. Free radicals are the bandits involved in many age-related disorders; they are unstable molecules that have lost an electron in the process of metabolism. Free radicals cause damage by stealing electrons from cells in nearly every tissue in the body. This damage can speed up the aging process, make it more difficult to fight off infection, lower defenses against heart disease, and damage DNA, which can lead to cancer.

As mentioned, free radicals are naturally created as the body performs basic metabolic functions. We do have repair mechanisms that can neutralize them, but our natural cleanup system can only do so much. Unfortunately, there are certain factors that place a terrible strain on the system—the environment and our chosen lifestyle. The environmental factors that stimulate free-radical production in our bodies include: UV rays, chemical radiation, cigarette smoke, automobile exhaust, and pesticides, to name a few. We also cause free radical damage by not getting enough rest or sleep, not managing our stress responses, not being physically active, and not eating healthfully. Vitamins A, C, and E are powerful antioxidants that help scavenge free radicals. Other antioxidants that provide protection against free radical damage include alphalipoic acid, selenium, and the carotenoids. These are readily available in fresh fruits and vegetables, but dietary supplements may still be necessary because the availability of nutrient-rich food has waned. You may want to visit our website to learn more about the dramatic impact that vitamins, essential fatty acids and amino acids can do to protect your health, emotional well-being, and mental functioning.

Putting Yourself on Your Priority List

Renée is a client who learned that many of the signs of advanced age that she experienced were due to neglecting proper nutrition, physical activity, and self-nurturing. As in so many other cases, her condition began to steadily improve once she reversed that neglect and put herself back on her priority list.

Renée's Story

Renée was a forty-one-year-old woman who had severe osteoarthritis of both knees. She initially visited the Institute for acupuncture as an alternative to surgery. The pain and swelling of her knees dramatically affected her quality of life. Renée was about forty pounds overweight and looked about fifteen years older than her age. There was a darkness to her eyes that, coupled with sagging jowls and a furrowed brow, made her seem depressed and weathered. In her initial consultation I found that Renée had taken care of a sick parent who passed away a year before our meeting. Before she could recover from that loss, her husband of eighteen years was diagnosed with a rapidly progressive neurological condition. At the time of my meeting with Renée, her husband was essentially homebound with very little use of his arms or legs. Renée had to bathe, clothe, and feed him, take care of the shopping and other household duties, and had very little time to attend to her own needs, or so she thought. As a result, her time for regular physical activity, proper nutrition, personal reflection, and recreation was gone. Renée never complained: she considered her role as caretaker to be paramount. But when the pain in her joints became severely limiting, she finally sought help.

Renée learned that her lack of exercise, depressed state, and poor nutrition had all contributed to premature aging and the worsening of her physical condition. The damage caused by such conditions is cumulative, we explained—but reversible. As Renée found, she could do many simple things for her body to boost its ability to fight premature aging, obesity, and joint problems. These included exercise, nutritional supplements, therapeutic massage, acupuncture, and counseling. Somehow, because we were doctors, our recommendations allowed Renée to start regarding these things as necessities rather than just self-pampering, and to make them a priority. Before long she joined our Obesity Treatment Group, which gave her the weekly support and encouragement she needed to shed pounds of the excess weight that had contributed to the destruction of her joints. She found that these protective, preventive, and reparative efforts also had cumulative results. Your body, too, will respond to these practices and provide you with additional proof of your amazing capacity for change.

Your life and well-being depend on the choices you make every minute of the day. This is not meant to impose an extra burden on your shoulders, but just to remind you that you were given life for a special purpose. Without taking proper care of yourself, you will not be able to fulfill your destiny. Treating these simple lifestyle adjustments as life-preserving habits will give you a renewed sense of purpose and an incredible sense of freedom. Rather than feeling deprived, you will feel like you are fully taking advantage of what life has to offer!

AFFIRMATIONS

*I will obtain regular health evaluations
to determine my baseline health
and fitness status.*

*I will become attuned to the messages of my
body that signal health and well-being.*

*I will heed the warnings my body sends to
alert me to problems in my physical condition.*

*I will begin to practice stress-relieving
techniques regularly.*

*I will increase my physical activity after
obtaining the "green light" clearance
from my health-care provider.*

*I will eat more balanced, nutritious
meals and snacks several times
each day, not late at night.*

*I will treat my body like a royal chariot,
with regular pampering and nurturing.*

The Plan

CHAPTER 5

Requirements:
Desire, Belief, and Dedication

Human beings have an amazing capacity for accomplishment and understanding. Our potential for achievement is limitless! We can accomplish nearly anything in life, whether health related or otherwise—as long as we have sufficient desire, belief, and dedication. These three key ingredients are absolutely necessary to achieve your simplest desires and your most lofty goals.

True *desire* comes from the spirit. When you feel an intense burning and yearning to live life fully, your spirit is engaged, and you are bound for heights of vitality. *Belief* rests with the mind and is closely linked to faith—whether you experience that as faith in a higher power, faith in the universe, or faith in that hidden part of yourself that will help you forge ahead even though your circumstances seem unfavorable. Your mind may acquiesce when your body is weak and tells you to give in, but you can overcome that inertia if you have a belief in your right and ability to reclaim wellness. Finally, you'll need *dedication* to keep yourself moving ever closer to your target and your body trained on its goal of vitality. Before we get into the five-step plan that will help you to start changing your life, let us examine these key attitudes in depth and guide you toward bolstering them, if necessary.

Desire

Without an intense desire to reach your destination, you may give up with the first sign of resistance. Therefore, before setting out on this new journey of living life to the fullest, ask yourself whether or not you *really* want it. Do you find that your wish for a better life keeps coming to you again and again? Do you find yourself talking about your desires constantly? If so, your desire is probably authentic. Desire is such a basic ingredient that I almost hesitate to bring it up. But many of my patients explain that their families, spouses, children, or society are pushing them into making certain health changes. They often agree to visit a doctor or health club just to get their loved ones off their backs—but they themselves don't really want to change. This is usually a prescription for failure, because they're not really committed. Inevitably, these individuals offer up halfhearted actions and wind up disappointed with their results.

Jack's Story

Jack was one such person. He never truly found a reason to live healthily. Though his lung cancer was caught in a fairly early stage he couldn't muster up the desire to modify his life. He wouldn't commit to change because, he said, after his second divorce he didn't have many positive elements in his life. Jack always seemed glum and pessimistic and did not bother to quit smoking until the cancer spread to his brain. Though it is tough to carry on in life when loneliness and depression set in, only the desire to live life fully can help you break free of limiting emotions and illnesses. You must have a *yearning* for wellness to spur you on.

Some people have an inner desire to be sick because they get certain benefits and special treatment. This desire is seldom conscious and can be tricky to overcome. Are you ready to give up some of the secondary gains you may have gotten from being sick, such as having someone else mow the lawn, do the laundry, or clean the house? Do you find that wallowing in self-pity has a greater pull for you than moving toward wellness? Are you sure you want to be well? If you really want to change your life for the better, you will do so. Be honest with yourself, because your own desire is a critical element for your success. Desire lays the foundation for the another ingredient: dedication.

Belief

In order to achieve, you must believe that achievement is possible. This is a critical step. Your belief is what first invites the universe to deliver to you everything you need to repossess wellness and achieve your personal destiny. Trust me when I tell you that you *can* reclaim wellness and live a fulfilled life, that the power already lies within your heart and soul. Your destiny has been with you from birth. You truly have a higher purpose in this world.

If doubt should creep into your consciousness, send it speedily on its way. Do not permit any reservations to linger; dispute them immediately. Repeat the affirmations at the end of this chapter and let them sink into your consciousness. Once they ring true for you, you will dispel doubt at every turn. Practice daily affirmation of the concepts outlined in this book and persevere in your pursuits.

State your desires out loud.

Envision yourself attaining them.

Embrace them as reality.

Do this faithfully, and the universe will assemble all of the necessary people, props, and details and send them flowing toward you. Tapping into your spiritual energy will provide you with answers to your questions and solutions to your health problems. Dare to believe! Everything that you need for your life's work and fulfillment will come to you. You will be fully capable of all the steps necessary to achieve your goals. Your faith will make it happen. With a sincere belief you can reach the heavens.

Catherine's Story

Catherine was a thirty-nine-year-old woman whose mother had died at the age of forty-five of a heart attack. Catherine had been devastated. Her mother never knew that she had heart disease. As a busy mom she did not regularly get health checkups or evaluations. She was also a heavy smoker and didn't exercise much. Her heart attack shocked the family.

Catherine knew that she had a genetic predisposition to develop heart disease at an early age. Nevertheless, she deeply believed that she could and *must* escape an early death due to heart disease. She pressed her medical doctor for suggestions as to what she could do to prevent the condition taking her life as well. She learned that clinical studies have shown that if a person at high risk for developing heart disease maintains a normal blood pressure and cholesterol level, exercises regularly, does not smoke, and gets routine health exams, they can dramatically lower their risk. She met other people in a support group who were also convinced that they had the power to change their fate, and they offered one another support and encouragement.

Catherine has been aggressive in her health regimen; she knows her life may depend upon it. She believes in her heart that her mother's early death was a warning that life is precious and that you must be informed of your health risks. She believes that her knowledge and faith will keep her alive to see her children graduate from college and possibly marry and have kids of their own.

Belief is a compelling force. Hold on to it and let it to propel you on your journey.

Dedication

Nothing worthwhile in life comes without effort. Yes, this is trite and even annoying, but it is the truth. Remember the old saying, Practice makes perfect? Mastering new skills and attaining new knowledge always—*always*—takes persistent effort. You will need dedication to persevere in the pursuit of wellness until it is attained. You must be willing to work through any pain or resistance to reach to the next level. Don't worry; this five-step plan will provide you with some tricks to keep you motivated and sticking to your plan.

A Lesson in Time Management

Now, you may say, "But Dr. Andrea, I don't have time to do all this stuff!" Think again. You cannot afford to skip anything; your very life depends upon it. You were not put here to live for household chores, errands, a job, or even only for your children. You must take the time to care for *yourself*. Otherwise the jobs you perform and the parental influence you demonstrate will only be halfhearted and counterproductive anyway. Properly caring for yourself, on the other hand, will make all of your work and errands easier and allow you more time to engage in your true purpose in life.

Imagine that I offered you a $60,000 shiny new convertible, fully loaded with all of the fancy options. Wouldn't you take the utmost care of it? No automatic car wash for *this* car: you'd likely clean and wax it by hand. And you certainly wouldn't allow your friends or children to eat or drink in it; they might soil the carpet or get rid of that new car smell. You would likely get the oil changed regularly and perform all the routine maintenance needed to keep this shiny new toy in tiptop shape, right?

Now suppose you had been out all day sporting around town in your new ride, and you found yourself low on gas. If I offered you a bottle of dirty water to put into the gas tank to get you home, would you pour it in? I don't think you would. You know that if you put anything other than gasoline into the gas tank, you will destroy the engine. And of course you know you'd have to spend thousands of dollars to get that engine back into working order.

Since our bodies serve to transport us through life in the same way, I am surprised how often people choose to abuse them by putting the equivalent of dirty water into their "gas tank," neglecting routine maintenance, or driving their body and mind to exhaustion. To make matters worse, there is no full-coverage insurance policy that will replace the body if it is abused or totaled in an accident. Yet most of us don't protect our bodies the way we would a mere automobile.

Making certain lifestyle changes does involve a bit of work in the beginning: there are no magic cures or instant prevention tricks. But have you considered the thousands of dollars you would spend on heart surgery? What about the cost of being removed from the fun and flow of life while recovering from a heart attack? Far better to take these simple little steps that I describe here. Taken together, they will bring a sort of magic into your existence that will make life worthwhile.

Michelle's Story

Michelle is a forty-five-year-old executive who visited the Pennington Institute for help in managing her high blood pressure. For the last eleven years, she explained, she had focused on her career, ignoring her personal health. She knew she had high blood pressure, but she never bothered to monitor it. Nor did she follow her healthcare provider's advice about managing her hectic and stressful lifestyle. She also neglected to get proper nourishment and exercise.

When Michelle was forty, her uncontrolled high blood pressure led to the onset of kidney disease. She was tied to a dialysis machine three times per week to purify her blood. She could no longer push herself to the limits she once endured, and her malfunctioning kidneys required her to make drastic changes in her diet. Michelle soon realized that taking an hour each week to shop for and prepare healthy foods, enjoying twenty minutes a day of regular physical activity, and taking little time-outs to pamper and nurture herself would have been quite reasonable prices to pay for the health she had taken for granted—and lost. She deeply regretted not doing something earlier. I beg you, do not follow in her footsteps. Live your life to the fullest in a balanced and functional way and make time for your health.

Please understand that success is not always attained through money or influential connections. Instead, the determining factors are belief, yearning, perseverance—and one more thing: accepting and embracing the idea that abundance and prosperity are available to all. Most of the successes our patients have enjoyed came through determination and dedication. They are people just like you: take strength from their tales of triumph, and rest assured that if they can reach their personal heights, you can do it, too. Your determination to move ahead will actually produce energy changes in your body. The power lies within you. You can attain the heavens; it's that simple. As long as you have the desire, belief, and dedication, you will succeed at living your destiny.

Do not equate past failures with your ability to succeed. Oftentimes our interpretation of past mistakes can make us think we're not capable of mastering new skills, completing new projects, or accomplishing our dreams. Perhaps when you last attempted to reach a certain goal, you did not yet have the skills necessary to master the task. Refuse to allow prior slipups and oversights to strip you of your confidence. Did you quit trying to walk as a toddler just because you fell flat on your face? Of course not. You cried a little, got right up, and tried again. Likewise, previous blunders and falls should not keep you from pushing toward your goals. You must *choose* to believe that your current intentions will have greater influence than your past failures. "That was then," you can say to yourself, "this is *now*." You have learned a great deal since then. You are even more curious and hungry than before; you are growing and experiencing life differently. Therefore, you are not doomed to repeat past errors.

Also remember that mistakes eventually lead to mastery. Our shortcomings can teach us what not to repeat, but they need not rob us of our self-assurance. On the contrary, they can stimulate us to strive even harder for excellence. This is where the mind can be our greatest ally or our nastiest adversary. It can boost us up or drag us down. So don't allow past troubles to get in your way. Learn from your mistakes, but don't dwell on them. Remember, you cannot reach back into yesterday to correct them, so it is useless to dwell on them. Holding on to the past can immobilize you. *You have the power, right now, to shape your future*. Let us find out how you can use that power wisely.

AFFIRMATIONS

Optimal health and well-being are my natural rights. I desire to reclaim wellness.

The ability to reclaim wellness is within me now. I believe in my power.

I know that mastery comes through repeated experience. I will continue to strive for excellence in everything I do. I am dedicated to my pursuit.

CHAPTER 6

Step 1: Define Your Goals

Now you have the foundation. You know that in order to reach your health and wellness goals, you must integrate your spirit, mind, and body. You have a sense of the part that each of these elements plays in your life, how each is meant to function, and what to do if you sense any *dys*function in them. And you understand the three personal characteristics required for success: desire, belief, and dedication. As you've probably noticed, the principles you've learned so far extend well beyond health and wellness: they are applicable to every area of your life, from family interactions and interpersonal relationships to self-mastery.

You are now well prepared to embark on the Pennington Plan, your five-step journey toward wellness. Each step of the plan will draw upon the different strengths inherent in your spirit, mind, and body and will help you to effectively incorporate them into your life. The steps will provide you with structure and guidance as you recondition your mind and body and welcome your spirit back into your life in ways you have likely forgotten. It will take time to retrain your body and reprogram your mind to act in wellness-promoting ways. Gaining control over your thoughts and behaviors and confidence in your spirit's guidance will take time as well. Nothing of value comes without effort, and habits are only formed with repetition. Gradually, however, you will find that you have fewer problems with doubt, frustration, and anger. The practices we'll discuss here will become automatic. You will become buoyant in attitude, stride, and physical condition and will naturally radiate a health and confidence that will transform your life. Let's learn more about how to implement the plan that will make your health goals a reality.

This chapter will map out the first step on the path to vitality: fully defining your goal. You will draw upon the power of your mind to create a clear vision of the new state of wellness that you aspire to. Through the practices outlined here, this blueprint will serve to mobilize the energy of your spirit and activate your whole physiology toward the achievement of your goal. Over time it will penetrate deeper, gradually becoming etched upon your subconscious as well.

Ask and It Shall Be Given

Have you ever seen a child whining and moaning as he tugs on his mother's skirt who, when asked what he wants, simply stares at her blankly, with no response? He probably just needs attention, of course, but you see how silly it would be to grumble about your circumstances without knowing what it is you want instead. The first step in defining your goal, then, is to ask yourself what it is you really want. What is your goal? How would you define it? What are the things you would change about your life or health? Does increased vitality, lower cholesterol, better blood sugar control, or a happy relationship interest you? Perhaps you simply want to wake up with a sense of peace and optimism. Just ask yourself these questions and welcome whatever comes to mind. Be adventurous and optimistic. Aim high! Remember, there are no limitations—unless *you* impose them.

Write It Down

The first step to achieving any goal is defining it as specifically and as simply as you can. So your assignment now is to record a precise description of your goal in your journal. Writing down an accurate depiction of your target will help to solidify and imprint it in your mind and heart. You will be taking it from the realm of obscurity to the realm of possibility and making it more tangible.

You may have several health goals, but start with one for now. As you become familiar with the process, you can do the same for others. Do not be discouraged or intimidated if your goal seems out of reach. Just putting it on paper brings it closer to existing in the physical realm—no matter how grandiose your goal may seem. Sometimes just writing your goal down shows you how attainable it is and how close you may already be to achieving it. It also helps to identify and demystify past hindrances to accomplishing it. When you see your goal in black and white, you will often learn that past blocks were only illusions, lacking any real substance.

Be very descriptive as you write down the elements that make up your wellness goal—just as if you were writing an entry for the dictionary. It's not necessary to use full sentences, but explain as best you can just what your wellness goal looks like. It may have been so long since you've been well that you don't even know what it would be like. In this case, you might start by answering a few questions.

Describe Your Well Self

In the next two sections you will devote yourself to imagining what it would be like if your health dream came true. Close your eyes and imagine that I wave a magic wand and magically transform you into the person you really want to be. Right now, at this very moment, you have achieved your goal. You are there! Count to five and open your eyes. Now, tell me: How does it feel to be you? How do you carry yourself now? How do you treat other people? How do other people treat you? How do you act in stressful situations? How do you spend your time? What is your outlook on life? What are your attitude and disposition like? What sorts of activities do you engage in? What new challenges are you going to tackle? What thoughts occupy your mind?

These questions will take some thought, but it is crucial to explore them thoroughly in your journal. What you are doing here is characterizing your "well self." Before you can see it happen in the physical world you must embrace your inner vision of the "new you" and mentally *become* that self. This goes beyond just saying that you won't have disease X or pain Y. It requires that you specifically affirm the values, qualities of personality, and type of character that you will embody. Are there people in your life or public figures who seem to have the disposition you aspire to attain? Watch what they do and how they speak, including their tone of voice and body language, to get a better sense of what you should focus on or emulate. Get a sense for the type of attitude and emotions you will display.

I believe that in order to resist those inner tendencies and outer circumstances that have disrupted your experience of wellness in the past, you need an accurate picture of the person you will be. By completely describing your well self, you can revisit your vision of what that self is like whenever you find yourself in an uncomfortable situation: your well self will help you get back on course. Here's an example from the journal of one of our clients:

Physical goal: *It is my intention to release 100 pounds.*

I am radiantly healthy. I see and experience my body as functioning properly and in a balanced manner. My skin is clear and glowing. My body is at its ideal weight of 138 pounds. I am energetic and enjoy a rich and full life because of it. I am confident and attractive. I see myself wearing beautiful and quality clothes that accentuate my fabulous figure. I speak about my experiences to others in order to support and inspire them to become healthy and fit. I often participate in physical events such as climbing, running, hiking, and 5 to 10K races.

This process of visualization worked well for a client of ours named Margaret, who was suffering from anxiety disorder. Her goal was to become a supervisor at her place of employment. She believed that she was qualified, but had some doubts about the other supervisors, who would have to approve the promotion. She felt that they didn't like her and would never help her advance in the workplace. Just thinking of asking for a promotion precipitated an anxiety attack. Her mind began racing; her heart was pounding and her palms sweating. She would even start feeling faint and nauseated.

Margaret's Story

As we began counseling with Margaret, we learned that her anxiety regarding the approval of her supervisor—or anyone of authority—stemmed from childhood experiences with her parents and three older sisters. Her older sisters excelled in math and sciences and seemed to receive all of the praise at the family dinner table. Margaret was more of a tomboy, enjoying basketball and track more than biology and geometry. Neither her sisters nor her parents supported her athletic pursuits, Margaret explained. They never attended track meets or playoff games or showed any interest in her sports; she never felt that she was smart enough to earn her parents' approval. Thanks to a couple of supportive teachers and coaches, however, Margaret still did well in both school and athletics. Their encouragement and praise kept her going all through high school.

Margaret's upbringing left her with what we call a negative, or pessimistic, way of explaining her world. She used to talk herself out of trying new things, engaging in a self-defeating internal dialogue that sounded very much like her parents' comments. When things got scary and she slipped into a panic attack, a voice inside her would say things like, "You're just not as good or smart as the others. What made you think you would succeed here?" On and on her internal monologue would run, pouring forth self-defeating statements that took away any faith she was holding on to. We told her that such a style creates its own reality, and encouraged her to start working on changing it. In his book *Learned Optimism*, psychologist Martin Seligman elaborates on the difference between optimists and pessimists. It turns out that people who are optimistic have characteristic ways of evaluating setbacks. They tend to attribute a problem or mishap not to their own ineptitude or incompetence but to factors outside of themselves—in other words, to temporary circumstances rather than permanent character flaws. By believing they will do better or be better prepared next time, they resist getting depressed or down on themselves. Through a number of research studies, Dr. Seligman has demonstrated that one way we can learn to become more optimistic is by changing the way we explain setbacks to ourselves. This in turn can make us both happier and more effective.

We asked Margaret to visualize herself at her goal, calmly sitting in the supervisor chair. See yourself handling the duties of your new position with the confident ability you know you possess, we said. We began with this visualization to stir up the positive self-beliefs implanted by her early life experiences with her teachers and coaches. Next we asked Margaret to visualize herself in the interview for the supervisor's position. Imagine yourself using your own positive energy to draw out the positive energy in your supervisor, we said. Imagine your supervisor responding to you in an encouraging way—more like your coaches in school and less like your parents. This rehearsal made Margaret calmer. When the time came for her interview, she excelled: she was relaxed and friendly and, with very little effort, got the promotion.

As you think about your goal from the standpoint of your well self, how will you talk to yourself about the challenges you face? Does your internal monologue typically include statements that are real downers? If so, change the dialogue. Flip it to be more supportive and encouraging. Find evidence to support your current goal by drawing strength from past successes:

> "I won that track meet last week; I can call on that same internal strength to beat this situation."

> "Just like the time I kept my promise to quit smoking when I was pregnant, I am going to take it one day at a time and stay true to my goal."

> "Okay, I didn't win last time. But I'm better prepared this time, and I am right for this position. I know I have what it takes to do this job. This time I'm going to win!"

Visualize Your Well Life

You have imagined the person you will be when your health dream comes true. Now imagine the life you will lead. Start by making a goal list. Jot down in your journal all the things you will do, all the experiences you want to have, as a result of realizing your goal. Imagine all of the activities you will engage in throughout the day. Imagine yourself interacting with others, both with people you know and total strangers.

Now close your eyes and take some time to see yourself living your dream. Create a mini-movie in your mind. Imagine yourself clearly in the picture, acting out every aspect that you detailed on your goal list. See your well self enjoying the goal in every way. If your goal is to have increased energy and enthusiasm for living, then visualize precisely how that feels. See yourself waking in the morning and greeting the day with an eager smile. Visualize yourself going about your morning routine with a spring in your step, with joy. See it all in crisp, rich detail. If you have ever felt the type of feeling you're aiming for, get in touch with the memory of that experience. Bring those memories to the forefront of your mind.

Here's a brief example of such a visualization that one client, Shelley, shared to help a group member who, like her, was suffering with depression. While her comrade was about to sink back into PLOMS (Poor Little Old Me Syndrome), Shelley offered her this lifeline from her journal:

> My goal: *To be happy and full of joy, free from depression*
>
> *What my goal looks like: I am smiling, I get out of the house and I connect with friends. I see myself laughing, I see sunshine and flowers, I hear the birds singing, and I walk with my head held high. I am carefree. I greet others with warmth and friendliness. I am embraced by loved ones. I hear the laughter of children.*

Did you notice how Shelley's description includes only positive images? Your goal description and visualizations should also be in the affirmative. They need to *inspire* you. Have you ever mentally rehearsed chewing somebody out, confronting a person who has done you wrong? If you have, you know that an imagined argument can flood your body with the same cascade of stress hormones as a real argument can. Here you're doing the opposite. Rather than imagining unpleasantness or misfortune, visualize and rehearse success.

Shelley said that meditating on these images and bringing them to life in her mind would actually make her smile. She would make an effort to smile at first, to shift her physiology and brain chemistry into happy mode. Soon enough, though, she found that her morning visualizations almost instantly brought a sense of inner joy and lightness. She would leave the house truly radiating warmth and kindness. And people would smile back at her! After a lifetime of depression this felt strange at first, she told us, but soon it began to seem natural to her. After following the plan and working with Dr. P in therapy for two months, Shelley broke out of the shell of depression that imprisoned her. These visualizations played a central role in setting her free.

The power to create lies within your imagination. Do not worry if you do not consider yourself to be a "visual person." You can still create a sense of how your dream-come-true will look and feel. If you can't see it in your mind's eye, then use words to describe how you'll behave or feel once you have reached the goal. Take it further and try to imagine what you will smell and hear. Will you cook yourself breakfast on the weekends? What will those eggs smell like? Will you have time for baths? How does that water feel? What lotions might you use? Will the phone ring more often? Who will be calling?

Make it real. Make it larger than life. Envisioning the realization of your goal will activate your personal power to manifest your desires. It will help you channel the organizing power of your mind to make your objective a reality. You will recruit vital energy that will stir your entire being into action. If you have physical limitations that would require miracles, you may decide to modify your dreams to those that seem "realistic." But don't be surprised if you achieve all your smaller goals and then some!

Stay Focused on the Goal and Release Self-Defeating Attitudes

That which you think, you are. By clearly imagining your accomplished goal, you will impress it into your physical reality. Focus on your healthy self-image several times a day—before getting out of bed in the morning and before falling asleep at night. Again, be specific about your goals and dreams. If you want to be well enough to run and play with your grandkids, then write down and visualize that outcome. Visualize the sights and sounds of the playground or soccer field, the beach, the family room. Refer to the goal list that you made above and visualize your health dream-come-true. Carry this list with you at all times and read the thoughts or images of the future goal to yourself many times throughout the day.

It is critical to keep focusing on the goal and *not* on the problems you must overcome. Obsessing over a problem only amplifies it in your life. Resist dwelling on the memory of past situations that are not helpful for the actualization of your goal. Those were the old you. Remember the biblical story of Lot's wife? Given the chance to escape certain death, she looked back with longing at her home and possessions and was turned into a pillar of salt. She never moved again. Looking back and focusing on the old you can make you stuck, unable to move forward.

How does your true, well self react to a slipup? Certainly it neither judges nor punishes you. Nor does it use the mistake as an excuse to throw in the towel and admit defeat. It is concerned only with learning from any mistakes, then releasing them and moving forward toward your future with confidence and peace. So let your mental pictures of your goal provide encouragement and reinforcement when you feel discouraged. Focus on your vision of the future and *not* on the limiting circumstance that you currently face. Remember to think of all that you will gain, rather than what you are giving up. Keep your eyes firmly fixed on the prize. Use your vision of wellness as much as you can to distract yourself from all of the pain or discomfort you may be experiencing. This is not to suggest that you should neglect a condition that is getting more painful or ignore the signals your body is giving you. In such cases you should seek treatment immediately. But once your condition is stable again, you simply must be sure that you are focusing on success—not on any negative experience or fears of failure.

Refer to your description often, visualize the end point, and be energized by it. As you announce and release your desires to the universe, an immeasurable exchange of energy transpires; before long you will manifest your goal in the here and now. Inventors and spiritual leaders throughout the ages have unleashed the great power that lies beyond the physical senses to reveal the secrets of science and the soul in the very same way. That same power is within you, and visualization is an excellent way to tap into it.

Live Like Your Well Self

Don't wait for your goal to be finally accomplished: start living the life of your well self *now*.

Rosa's Story

One of our clients, Rosa, had a goal to lose weight: seventy-five pounds of it. Rosa had been a beautiful, vibrant, and outgoing woman—that is, until she married her first husband. He adored her exuberance when they first met, she said, but once they were married, he became insecure about her alluring figure and outgoing personality. She had always dressed tastefully, but he soon discouraged her from wearing short skirts or showing too much of her body. He gave her a hard time whenever one of his friends remarked how attractive she was. Unable to tolerate his nagging, she soon began putting on weight, hiding her vivacious persona and physical attributes. She felt much less feminine, but it helped to stop her husband from making her feel like a "tramp." After four years of this abuse, Rosa divorced him— but the negative treatment continued. He made her feel as though she would never be a good mother to their only child. He was so convincing, she said, that her subconscious mind soaked it all up. Whenever she thought someone was admiring her, her subconscious would deliver up nasty little phrases in his voice: "They don't care about you; they just want your body. What kind of mother cares what others think of her looks?" He had her convinced: a good wife and a good mother couldn't be alluring. Rosa lost her self-confidence and self-love for quite some time.

Following the plan, however, she began visualizing herself at her reduced weight and size. As she began to explore the specific elements of her goal in her mind, Rosa found that merely being thinner was not enough. As she put it: "I want to put the *va* back in my *voom!*" Her vision went beyond the physical; she saw its emotional and spiritual dimensions as well. She wanted to embody a whole new attitude and spirit, one that was as lively and vivacious as she once had been. When the dietary restrictions and physical training got rough for her, Rosa would visualize the bright countenance and demeanor that she had in her twenties and early thirties, before the birth of her first child. Rather than dwell on her resistance to her new meal plan and fitness regimen, she focused all of her energies on the positive outcome. The practice of visualizing her alluring figure, "vavoom!" attitude, and hopeful mindset helped her to stay motivated and stick to her new lifestyle plan.

Most significantly, the visualizations of her future self prompted Rosa to begin enacting her health dream *while in the process* of losing weight. She didn't wait for the complete attainment of her weight-loss goal. She challenged herself to engage in all of the behaviors of her slimmer, future self. She made eye contact with people she passed on the street. She allowed herself all sorts of pampering and self-nurturing: rich bubble baths, romantic dinners for one, little love notes to herself. When offered invitations to events that required walking or being physical, Rosa didn't make excuses—she went, and behaved as though she was at her ideal weight, rather than sitting self-consciously in the corner. This part of the plan helped to keep her motivated, lifted her mood, and mobilized an energy that she hadn't felt since her early adult years. She started to carry herself with greater confidence and optimism. She soon found herself in the zone, no longer fighting resistance. She found her stride and excelled! She tapped into the self she once was even before she'd lost all the weight she'd gained and found that people began to see her joyful, well self as the person she really *is*.

Living this way, Rosa realized, had always been a matter of choice: her well self had always existed within. Rosa was empowered to make the choice of looking beyond her overweight condition and beyond the emotional trauma that she had been carrying around in the locked chest of her subconscious. She concentrated on the new, true Rosa, embraced her higher self, and started living again!

Fake It Until You Make It:
The Power of Make-Believe

As a child, you created magic with your imagination—effortlessly! Your natural capacity for role-playing allowed you to fly through space in the rocketships of your mind. There's absolutely no reason why, as an adult, you cannot utilize the amazing tool of make-believe to deal with any situation that you would otherwise find difficult or unpleasant, as we shall see. First, however, I am not recommending here that you attempt to force from your mind any situation that truly requires emotional healing time. If you find that you are dealing with an issue that is particularly painful, and you think that you may need therapy or counsel, do not hesitate to get attention and support. Do not deny yourself the grieving process if you've lost a loved one. Make-believe is meant not to replace these healing processes but to offer you a wonderful coping mechanism—a very effective one, and one that opens you up to truly take advantage of this five-step plan.

If you can't start living the life of your well self now, in actuality, do so in your mind. If you start feeling down or like you just can't make it, come back to your written description of your goal and make believe that you have achieved its full realization. This will motivate you to pick yourself up and keep going. Reliving negative or stressful experiences in your mind or in conversation can only stir up negative energy and drain all the life out of you. Certainly you've felt the anger or self-pity well up inside when you're telling someone else about your bad day or getting sensitive issues off your chest. This can put your physiology back into "sad" or "mad" mode, causing a release of stress hormones.

Instead, let your well self tell the story. Use make-believe to keep your cool. You may have already seen this in action. Have you ever seen someone tell about a day in which everything went wrong—but with a big smile on their face, as if all their mishaps and misadventures were just part of a joke? You can do the same. Think about it: your vibrant, well self would never be thrown by these experiences. So if you feel you must tell someone about a miserable experience you've just endured, imagine telling it in the voice of your well self. Tell the story as if it were so light and comical that it *had* to be something out of a movie. This will keep you in an upbeat mood and won't depress your entire physiology with stress hormones.

Betsy's Story

Make-believe helped Betsy, a patient of ours suffering with fibromyalgia. Betsy spent a great deal of time in bed because of extreme fatigue and muscle pain. She knew that if she would only engage in *some* activity she would get moderate relief from her pain and weakness. But besides her physical pain, getting out of bed was also a serious mental challenge. Though her brain said "do it," her will said "forget it." I taught her to use make-believe in these situations. In her visualizations, Betsy had told me, her well self didn't make excuses; she pulled herself up and got going—with a smile. So I recommended that she engage in an imaginary self-monologue from the perspective of her well self. Talk to yourself out loud if necessary, I said, to kick-start your willpower. Betsy's suggested self-chat, in a perky, optimistic voice, went something like this:

> Okay, Betsy, the sun is shining and we've got to get moving! Physical activity brings such joy and energy that it's worth every ounce of effort. Now, Betsy, you are such a lovely person that the world needs to see you for at least an hour today. So get your beautiful self out of bed. Let's go! No excuses, dear. Life is for the living and moving, so let's move! Let's live!

"Speak these words to yourself with optimism and a smile," I told her, "and get out of bed as if you *were* the well self that you visualized."

This is silly, Betsy thought at first. I can't do this. I explained that if she would just fake it internally and at least get started externally, she could get over the initial hump of resistance and sail on from there. After a week, Betsy found that she was not only able to get out of the bed, but out of the house as well, and for more than an hour. She found that her inner cheerleader was always there. It did take considerable conscious effort to silence the chatter of her normal, pessimistic, weaker self and switch on the monologue of her perky well self. But she found that it was worth the effort. It became infectious: she began using this technique in other areas of her life. Betsy told us that through make-believe she got her *real* life back.

This technique works particularly well when you know exactly what you want to do—in Betsy's case, get out of bed and start moving—but don't have enough motivation to start doing it. If you allow your inner cheerleader to motivate you to engage in one of the things that you *know* will get you closer to your goal, even for just an hour, you will see results. Remember, though the journey may be a thousand steps long, each step inevitably brings you closer to your destination.

I use make-believe myself whenever I get into a bad mood. Sometimes things can really get under my skin. Perhaps you can relate to this scenario: you've got an early-morning flight scheduled and you set your alarm clock, but of course it doesn't go off. Instead, you're awakened by the sound of the garbage truck barreling down your street. Naturally, you didn't put the trash out the night before: you intended to do that in the morning on your way out. You rush to shower and get ready, then snag your stockings on the way out of the door—or, if you're a man, you nick yourself shaving *three* times. As you hustle to leave the house, you kick over the dog's water bowl. Of course you have to fill it up. The taxi to the airport keeps blowing the horn, as if you don't already know that you'll miss your plane if you don't leave soon. After all that frustration you arrive at the airport, in a foul mood but in the nick of time—and your flight is canceled!

A similar scenario happened to me not long ago. Due to a flight cancellation, I got to a speaking engagement on the West Coast a day late and without my luggage. As I sat on the airplane, tired and disgusted and feeling sorry for myself, I began to think about the power of the mind and how imagination can affect our mood and performance. I knew that if I went into the conference in a low mood, the audience would pick up on it: the energy would be all wrong, and I'd likely do a poor job. So, I decided I would try to flip things around, to whisk the bad mood away with a make-believe "perfect trip." I decided to imagine that everything in the cross-country flight had gone amazingly *well*. What would that be like? Well, I imagined that I sat in first class, of course, and heard all of my favorite leisure-time songs. (I even began to hum my favorite tunes with a smile on my face as if I were perfectly cool, calm, and collected, which was still far from the case.) I wasn't put up in a dingy hotel without my suitcase, toothbrush, or change of clothes. No, they took me to a five-star hotel, where I woke to a hot luxurious bath, a deluxe room-service breakfast, and a plush limousine ride back to the airport. Nothing to stew about there! It took some mental gymnastics, but I began to act as though the unexpected layover were a planned part of my journey. I visualized the attitude, demeanor, and internal calm I would have if I'd had the perfect journey. I began to imagine myself walking into the conference with a radiant smile on my face, in my very casual travel wear (jeans, tennis shoes, and a sweatshirt!), as if this were the original plan. I specifically avoided imagining myself sulking during the meeting or groveling for forgiveness from the conference organizers as if I were a puppy who'd just been scolded for chewing on her master's slippers.

This attitude, though make-believe at first, started to diffuse through my being like sunshine through the clouds. I radiated such a warmth and confidence at the conference that the attendees thanked and congratulated me for injecting energy and enthusiasm into the meeting. The rest of my trip fell into place just as smoothly. It was amusing at the time, but it proved to me the amazing power we have at our disposal to consciously mold any situation into the reality we desire.

You will no longer be a victim of your emotions or circumstance as long as you focus your imagination and energy wisely. No matter the mental or physical obstacle, you can call forth energy, emotions, and physical strength to make your goal real. Be specific in your description of your wellness goal—whether it is your goal of the hour, as in my example above, or of a lifetime—and diligent with your daily visualizations of it. Define it. Imagine it. Focus on the positive image often. As you go into your meditations or as you walk through nature, imagine that you *are* the person in your image. Let go of the past; let go of draining emotions. Be the well self that you've imagined in you mind—right now.

AFFIRMATIONS

*I will clearly define my goal and
visualize it several times each day.*

*I will embrace the attitude, demeanor,
and emotions of my well self.*

*I will focus on my goal at all times and
not allow my current problems to rob
me of my confidence or enthusiasm.*

CHAPTER 7

Step 2: Define Your Motivations

By now you've thoroughly explored your wellness goal. You've visualized the person you'll be and the life you'll lead. You know *what* you want to achieve. But why? What are your motivations for reaching that wellness goal? This seems like such a simple question, but I ask it for good reason. I want you to come up with five factors that will motivate you to reach the goal you described in Step 1—five reasons that living well is important to you. Write them down in your journal. Doing so will be critical to your success with this plan, for two reasons. First, because thinking deeply about your reasons and motivations will give you an even better understanding of what brought you to this point and why moving forward is so important. Second, because it will bind you even more strongly to success. When things get tough, and sometimes they will, you'll need to dig deep inside and focus on exactly why you want to achieve your dream. Having thought deeply about your motivations—and having your list of them nearby—will help to keep you on track.

For instance, suppose your goal is to quit smoking. Why? "Well, everyone knows smoking is bad for you. I don't want to end up with lung cancer or emphysema." This is an excellent reason, certainly, one that can carry you along for quite a while. But one day you're going to feel so frenzied and frazzled that you'll be sorely tempted. The possible consequences seem so distant; surely a few puffs won't do any harm? After all, you might die from some other cause long before cancer sets in, right? You know deep down that those puffs could put you right back where you started, but the risk of some far-off illness might not be enough to help you resist the temptation.

Once you explore your motivations seriously, though, you realize you have other reasons, too. Cancer and emphysema are not the only health risks: smoking raises the risk of heart disease and a whole host of other conditions as well. You want to be active without panting. You want to create a healthier environment for your children. You resent all the money you're spending on a habit that isn't even good for you. And you *hate* having to huddle outside a building, cupping that cigarette on a cold winter day. Remembering all your reasons for quitting may tip the scale: you may be able to throw the cigarettes away and choose a diversion instead. Those extra motivations can help you fight temptation and win.

What do you value most? Are you pursuing your goal to ensure that you'll be around to see your children grow up, go to college, get married, and have children of their own? Maybe you just want to function with less pain. Or perhaps you'd like to revive your vitality so that you can travel with your partner and explore distant places together. Maybe you'd like to learn more, grow more, experience more in general. Is it primarily for yourself that you want to accomplish your dream? Or is it for your family, or your mate? Be as honest as you can: there are no good and bad reasons, only more or less powerful motivators. As you list your motivating factors, you may discover that you have been neglecting your health at the expense of what—or who—is most important to you. Most of us don't take the time to really think about what we value most in life, but doing so will make all the difference in sticking to your wellness plan. So whatever your motivations are, list them. No apologies are necessary. Do not make any excuses for your desires. There should be no guilt associated with your motivations to live better and enjoy life. That's why you're here; you deserve it!

As in the example above, your motivations can include not only things you want to enjoy but also illnesses or conditions you want to avoid. Usually focusing on a positive image of the future is most inspiring, but considering the consequences of *not* following your plan may work better for you. Are you motivated to begin a wellness plan to prevent a heart attack? To keep yourself from falling deeper into a pit of depression? To escape the clutches of an addiction? To give yourself a body you're not ashamed of? Sometimes thinking of all the things that could happen to you if you *don't* change your life can help propel you onto the path toward emotional stability and physical vitality. So whether you are driven by the pursuit of joy or the avoidance of pain, list five motivating factors that you can rely on to keep you moving toward your goals.

You may wonder why you need five reasons. Why not four, or six? You can certainly list more or fewer if you want, but five just seemed like the perfect number to us: enough to keep you motivated in different situations, but not too many to remember easily and tick off on the fingers of one hand. Think about it: each of your five fingers has properties that make it more useful for certain tasks than others. You could manage with fewer—or more—but it's easiest to grasp things, write, and perform other tasks when all five are present. Similarly, depending on your changing mood and circumstances, you may need several different motivating factors. They can all work together to keep you on your path.

Anthony's Story

For instance, Anthony, a divorced father of three, was dreading his treadmill workouts. So we asked him to think of his top motivating factors and to begin to visualize himself at his goal enjoying them. He listed his top motivators for getting in shape this way:

- *To play more actively with my children*

- *To feel more confident about my looks and appearance*

- *To be able to be active without stopping to catch my breath*

- *To be able to be active with greater mobility and fewer joint problems*

- *To look better in a bathing suit*

Anthony began to imagine himself already having the things he was working so hard for: looking slim and fit at the beach with his kids, playing with the kind of energy they had without gasping for breath. He saw himself laughing and relaxed, acting with new confidence, no longer being shy. The thought of attaining these things often kept him going five more minutes on the treadmill, burning off more calories. If he felt too tired or bored to go on, he'd encourage himself to go just one minute more for each of his three boys. Over time, as his cardiovascular condition improved, he noticed that his workouts got easier. He had more energy and became more determined than ever to stick with the program. His motivating factors made all of his hard work begin to seem like child's play.

Rate Your Motivations

Now that you have investigated your reasons for your wellness goal, I want you to rate each of your motivating factors. Quantify how badly you want it. Give each motivator a number from 1 to 5, where 1 represents the lowest motivation and 5 the highest. How important is your heart, your peace of mind, or your quality of life? For a desired outcome, use the following value scale:

> 5—I have a burning desire for this. This goal made me commit to the Pennington Plan.
>
> 4—I definitely want to achieve this and am willing to put in serious effort to do so.
>
> 3—This would be a nice fringe benefit to have as well.
>
> 2—I don't care about this so much myself, but it's important to those around me.
>
> 1—My mind knows this is good for me, but my heart really isn't in it.

Use this value scale to rate an outcome you want to avoid:

> 5—I'm really scared of this, and I'll do anything I can to avoid it.
>
> 4—I certainly don't need this in my life, and I'm willing to devote serious effort to preventing it.
>
> 3—I'd rather avoid this if possible.
>
> 2—This doesn't really trouble me, but it bothers those around me.
>
> 1—My mind knows this is bad for me, but my heart doesn't really believe it.

Quantifying your motivation and desire will give your plan for change a strong driving force. It will help shape and channel the energy that you bring to transforming your life. You will know what is most important to you and what is less important but still desirable. The motivations with a score of 4 or 5 will stir up the greatest amount of inner strength and power. They are the ones you will come back to most often to keep moving forward, the ones that will keep you going when you feel like quitting. The lesser-ranked motivators may not be able to carry your efforts alone, but they can certainly contribute to your overall motivation and help fill out the picture.

When you're feeling weak, concentrate on as many of your motivating factors as necessary to help you resist the temptation to retreat or resign. You may find, too, that your ratings evolve over time—that something you once viewed as merely a nice fringe benefit becomes so rewarding as to merit even more serious effort. (A word of caution: If at any point you find that none of your motivations really ranks a 4 or a 5, consider choosing another goal, something you want more strongly. Without a burning desire, you are more likely to fall off the wagon; you are likely to need at least one 4- or 5-ranked reason to accomplish anything transformative.)

I know that the conditioning of the mind is tough to change. It's easy to fall prey to the reflexive negativity and bad habits that have made themselves your constant companions. But you *do* have the power to achieve your health dream, and now you can more consciously draw upon your motivations to activate that inner strength. Focusing on your motivating factors will stimulate every cell in your body to make your health goal a reality. Consciously directing your mental energy will produce tangible results on the physical plane. And knowing all the reasons you've been wanting it so badly will make the victory all the sweeter.

AFFIRMATIONS

*I will ask myself what I truly value
in life and define my motivations
for embracing wellness.*

*I will focus on my motivating factors
and allow them to inspire me when
my resolve weakens.*

*I will use the vision of myself enjoying my
motivating factors to keep me on course.*

*I will carry my list of motivators with me
and review them, one by one, whenever
I need to renew my enthusiasm.*

CHAPTER 8

Step 3: Devise a Plan and Get Started!

You can't be expected to easily navigate a course from Los Angeles to Washington, D.C., without a road map. In the same way, you need a practical plan that will guide you to your wellness destination. You are changing over from the fast lane of bad habits to the health-promotion highway; you need a strategy that offers guidance and structure but is flexible and adaptable. To ensure maximum results, your health plan should include components for boosting the health and vitality of all the elements of your being: mind, body, and spirit. As you engage these elements in your plan and your life in general, you will notice that improvements in one area will strengthen and heighten the effectiveness of the others. Your whole being will become better integrated. This chapter gives some guidelines to help you create and act upon your personal plan for improving your health and living the life you've always wanted.

List Five Pathways to Your Goal

There are usually several acceptable ways to get from point A to point B. Any number of possible roads can lead to your health destination, and we do not want to get locked into one method or strategy. Having only one approach can often make us feel limited or trapped and only leads to disappointment if the original course becomes unworkable. So I want you to set yourself up for success by outlining at least *five* pathways to your goal. Based on your health and the specific goal you have in mind, which practices will help you to achieve it? Make a list of them in your journal. This step will get your creative juices flowing and mobilize your energy for change. If you cannot think of five pathways, leave one or more labeled as "other." By doing this you will remain open to the infinite possibilities that exist beyond your current perception and allow the universal intelligence to offer alternative paths to your goal in the future.

Of course, given the questions we have already explored, you may have more than five ways in mind to increase your vitality. You may quickly come up with several practices for mental well-being and clarity, several more for physical vitality, and a couple of ways you might attain spiritual peace. So while I suggest that you come up with five, I do not intend that you become fixed on these as the *only* possible roads: you may find yet another or *many* other avenues that may actually be more appropriate. But outlining five methods will be more than enough to get you going.

Elements of a Successful Health Plan

As you devise your plan, be sure to address each part of your nature—spirit, mind, and body. As you learned earlier, this will help you draw upon your inherent strengths and fully realize your health potential. Though it's tempting to focus on one major area, you will find that you are brought closer to the enjoyment of your goal when every part of your nature is involved in the process. Begin to integrate physical activity with more introspective spiritual pursuits and more outwardly directed mental exploration.

Gayle is a fifty-two-year-old woman who wanted a complete overhaul of her life: health, habits, relationships, and career. She told us that the stress of her job and her children leaving home for college was wreaking havoc on her eating habits and her marriage, and that her energy for self-nurturing and self-development had been whittled away to nothing. We began with a focus on her weight-loss goals as she worked through the more sensitive issues with Dr. P. Here is what her wellness plan looked like:

Goal: To be a healthy weight, with a BMI below 25		
	MIND	**BODY**	**SPIRIT**
1.	don't worry	eat healthful, whole foods	pray
2.	reduce stress	increase physical activity	let go, let God
3.	talk with friend	walk with friend	worship with friend
4.	keep learning	drink more water	laugh out loud
5.	think positive	get facials, massages	do the right things

Note that Gayle's goal seems at first to pertain only to her body. But, again comparing the human body to an automobile, how do you maintain a healthy relationship to your car? Well, you don't want that relationship to consist solely of *you* taking care of *it*; you want *it* to take care of *you* as well! You know that for optimal performance you need to give it adequate fuel and regular maintenance. But it can't sit around in the garage all the time. Your car should not only take you to work, school, and on errands, but on drives in the country and out for some adventure as well. Similarly, your overall plan should move you beyond mere preoccupation with repairs and overhauls to an existence that is rich with experience and that inspires you to laugh, love, create, and explore:

- Our bodies perform best when we are moving: include adequate physical activity as part of your plan. (Remember to consult your health-care professional to determine which activities are most appropriate for your situation.)

- Our minds perform best when exercised and stimulated: include exploration and learning as part of your plan.

- Our spirits soar with delight when engaged in the expression of our innermost desires and talents: include the activities that truly express your spirit as part of your plan.

- Body, mind, and spirit perform best when allowed proper rest, relaxation, and freedom from stressful situations: include stress-reduction techniques and seven to nine hours of sleep each night as part of your plan.

- Our entire being functions optimally when nourished with proper fuel: include healthy, nutritious meals and plenty of water as part of your plan. (Check with your health-care provider to see whether nutritional supplements may be appropriate for you, especially if you are facing a chronic disease or deficiency.)

For optimal health and vitality, each of these should be part of your everyday regimen, just as they were in your childhood. Early childhood is probably the closest many of us got to the balanced, integrated life that we all need to embrace for total life fulfillment and optimal health. So inject a childlike sense of adventure into your life.

Embrace an outlook of creativity and wonder and make some plans for living life to the fullest.

Set Milestones
Without Time Constraints

If your goal is likely to take months or years to attain, be sure to set achievable milestones along the way. Otherwise, you may become tired, frustrated, or discouraged, thinking—mistakenly—that you're not making any progress. Establishing mini-goals to reach for along the way demonstrates progress much more clearly. For instance, if your goal is to reduce the number of cigarettes you smoke from twenty per day to zero, you should set some milestones that you can observe—down to ten, down to five—and celebrate. (You'll learn more about this in the fourth step of the plan.) This will help you recognize that though your final goal may still be a fair distance away, you are making significant progress. You will become more confident that you have what it takes to reach your goal and be inspired to even further effort.

Imposing rigid time lines on ourselves can make us tense or discouraged if we don't achieve our goal by the designated time. Don't be too hard on yourself if reaching even your interim milestones takes longer than you thought. Some goals, such as lowering your cholesterol or losing weight to avoid a heart attack, certainly justify a businesslike approach or even some sense of urgency. In general, however, you should not allow yourself to feel pressured by the time it takes you to reach your goal. Science shows us that putting unnecessary pressure on ourselves will only rev up the nervous system and stress us out. This can deplete the brain's serotonin and dopamine stores. Remember that these brain chemicals are linked to mood, energy level, and motivation. Having decreased levels of these chemical messengers, which happens when we are chronically stressed, can lead to depression, low energy, and a feeling of defeat.

This is not a fad plan for short-term returns only; you should view this as a lifestyle guide that you will continue to refine with experience. If you do set a target date for achieving your goal, be easy on yourself. Pressure is healthy to the degree that it serves to gently keep you on task, but don't let it frustrate you or rob you of your drive and enthusiasm. Take each day as it comes and make the best of it. If you find yourself missing the target, you may need to readjust your aim and your expectations. Remember, you're doing this to get more *joy* out of life, not more pain. So don't torture yourself. If you like, avoid setting time limits on the attainment of your goal altogether, and just remember that each step you take brings you closer to it. Your journey will involve making many lifestyle changes that, taken together, will ensure your success. So, stick with your plan and keep moving. Enjoy the process and take comfort in knowing that you are on your way to increased vitality and bliss. You are doing something worthwhile and beneficial, and there is absolutely no need for self-abuse.

Reprogram the Subconscious Mind for Success

Creating a road map toward greater health and well-being includes not only selecting new behaviors and steps that will take you there but also letting go of the ones that hindered your progress before or caused your dis-ease in the first place. As explained in Chapter 3, many of the illness-promoting behaviors we engage in are automatic, prompted by diverse psychological and environmental cues. A lifetime of conditioning leads us to unconsciously respond to these cues with certain predictable habits. Remember, it is your subconscious programming that leads to your reactions. Think of reactions as simply *repeated* *actions*, things you have done so often that you now do them automatically, unconsciously, and without thinking.

For instance, many of us have conditioned ourselves, over time, to eat while entertaining or in social settings, snack while watching TV, have a cigarette or a drink in response to stress, and consume large amounts of unhealthy "comfort food" in response to sadness or anxiety. Once your subconscious has been programmed, it can be hard to resist the impulses that these cues trigger—*but you can*, when you are prepared for them.

To reprogram your subconscious, you must first identify the triggers that lead to the behavior you want to change. In the examples above, parties, watching television, stress, and anxiety are all triggers. Once you realize and remember that, you can begin to uncouple them from the unhealthy behaviors they lead to. This involves making a conscious decision to resist your automatic, unconscious reactions. To break the association, you must have a healthy response in mind that you will perform instead of the detrimental preprogrammed behavior. In the examples above, we find that watching TV is a cue that triggers unhealthy snacking. You could uncouple the association of TV and snacking by simply not snacking, or you could create a new associated link by repeatedly engaging in a new activity with the TV stimulus. For example, rather than snacking, choose to exercise instead. Charge yourself an exercise "entry fee" for watching your favorite TV show. Take a walk before the big football game or movie, ride the stationary bicycle while watching the show, or do sit-ups and push-ups during every commercial break. In this way you will uncouple the TV trigger from the behavior of eating unhealthy snacks.

Make no mistake: at first this will feel downright unnatural, even silly. After all, you're trying to uncouple a habit that was years in the making. The first time you actually choose that new, healthy activity over that old bad habit is always the most difficult of all. The second hardest is doing it again. Sooner or later, though, it will start to become easier every time. In the example above, the more consistently you exercise before or while watching TV, the stronger the new association will become. The more times you avoid the old, preprogrammed behavior (eating while watching TV), the less potent a trigger for unhealthy snacking the TV trigger becomes. After a while you will find that watching TV just doesn't *feel* right without some sort of physical activity to go with it. To help yourself stick with the new behavior (in this case, exercise), focus on your motivations for eliminating the bad habit. Reinforce the new activity in your mind by consciously reviewing the ultimate benefits. Soon, you won't even *think* of giving in and forfeiting all that you've gained. This may take you some time to accomplish, but it *does* work.

You can use the same method to reprogram your responses to stress. Once you consciously recognize the stressful situation as a possible trigger, you can choose to stretch, sing, go for a fast walk, or pamper yourself with a bubble bath rather than reaching for a smoke or booze. The more times you give up the old behavior, the more its power to tempt will fade away. Dr. P said that she used to clean her house to dispel frustration or anger instead of keeping them bottled up inside. That way, by the time the feeling passed she not only had resisted doing something she would regret but also had a clean house.

Instead of centering social events around food, center friendly get-togethers around sharing and experiencing life, laughter, and love. How? Get caught up on one another's lives while enjoying a walk through the park or a hike in the woods. Share your interests by visiting a museum or art gallery. If you must entertain around meal or snack time, encourage your guests to bring healthy items and experiment with desserts that are not loaded with tons of fat and sugar.

Once you identify your triggers, you can take a multipronged approach to reprogramming your subconscious for success using some of the techniques you've learned in this book. For example, if sadness regularly triggers you to binge on candy or cakes, the first step to take is not to buy them. Buying sweets would be a setup for defeat, not success. Eliminate the possibility of engaging in the behavior at all by not allowing it a place in your home or workplace. This is what we call taking control of your environment: by doing so, you reduce or eliminate the possibility of being tripped up by pitfalls.

Second, make a list in your journal of five possible actions you could take in response to the depression rather than reaching for food. One of our clients wrote them down like this: . .

In the past I have given in to binge snacking when I get depressed and anxious by my workload or my home situation. Instead, if I get upset . . .

1. I will retreat to a quiet place and take five deep breaths to get centered.

2. I will stretch or take a brisk walk to dispel the negativity.

3. I will call a friend for support.

4. I will say a prayer or affirmation.

5. I will work on letting go of the emotion in the moment and change my focus to something uplifting.

Stick to your new solutions by thinking of the consequences of the old action and focus on the benefits you'll enjoy by choosing the new ones instead.

Finally, I also suggest that you use the techniques described in Chapter 2 to get in touch with and dispel the negative emotions so that you are not driven by them at all.

Once you recognize and acknowledge your temptations, you will be primed for success. I promise you that as you consciously take control of your actions, you will prevent the nagging dragons of your past from keeping you from your destiny. You will expose them for the illusions that they are and strip your prior weaknesses of their power to undermine your efforts. Remember this: Your inner essence cannot be attacked or denied. Your true self does not need the approval of others. It is whole and secure in itself, just as you are.

Foresee Pitfalls

Would a long-distance cyclist begin a seventy-mile bike ride through the countryside without an adequate water and nutrient supply? Certainly not. He knows that as he treks through the heat he will be losing water that must be replenished. And his muscles will not support him without sufficient nutrient replacement. The success of his journey, therefore, depends upon proper planning. If you were navigating a course through the mountains, you would need to anticipate the weather and be aware of the terrain to prepare for the driving conditions. You might need to put special snow tires on your vehicle. If the road is likely to be too dangerous for nighttime driving, you would need to map out places to rest along the way. In much the same way, you need to anticipate the situations you will encounter on your road to health.

As they embark on a new journey toward wellness and reprogramming the subconscious, I encourage all of my patients to prepare for success by foreseeing pitfalls and planning for the tough times. This makes the journey as foolproof as possible. If you're going on a long car trip, for instance, you know that your dining options along the way will be limited; you're going to have a hard time resisting the temptation to pick up some fast food as soon as you get hungry. So if you're trying to eat healthfully, don't get on the road unprepared: make a trip to the grocery store for wholesome snack items *before* leaving town. Determine to be successful with proper preparation, as in the following formula: *Combine 2 parts determination with 2 parts preparation 4 success!*

Preparing for pitfalls ahead can extend well beyond travel and food. This principal is absolutely critical, for example, not only in the treatment of addictions but in programs designed to teach people how to overcome any destructive habits. Previously, I asked you to face up to your "issues." Are there internal obstacles that you've faced before that you can expect to encounter again? I bet there are. Lifestyle change is *always* accompanied by challenges. It is best to acknowledge right up front any personal weaknesses or temptations that may present themselves as pitfalls on your journey. Jeffrey weighed over 500 pounds when he came to us, and he was determined to lose weight. But he also had considerable insight into the mental pitfalls that might beset him along the way. Here is the way he described them:

My pitfalls from reaching my "well self" are as follows:

1. I tend to self-sabotage myself. Maybe I believe the sabotage is repayment for some disobedience of the past.

2. My lack of discipline comes from working really hard for something and being disappointed (i.e., I have a master's degree, I am going for a doctorate, and it has been really difficult to obtain decent employment. I only had a respectable, paying job for one month, and I have either been underemployed or hustling for money). I tend to be apathetic because I feel the fruits of my labor won't pay off.

3. Because I can mess up, I think I am disqualified to help others, so I may stay imprisoned at my own "pity party."

4. I have *never* been thin, and it irritates me that people would show me more love and respect just because I was thinner. The militant and defiant part of me will want to be big just for the purpose of people discriminating (they have no right!).

5. I can be really concerned about what people say, and if I hear something hurtful, it can throw me off, or I give up.

Denial not only delays success but also has the power to sabotage your efforts. As you begin to overcome urges, change long-standing habits, or disable certain prompters, set yourself up for success by planning to address them head-on. What are your pitfalls? Have stressful situations prompted binge eating, substance abuse, or social withdrawal in the past? Have feelings of low self-esteem, ineptitude, or lack of determination prevented you from sticking with past health regimens? Perhaps you have projected hostility or responded defensively when challenged, and this sent you into an emotional tailspin. By examining past obstacles, internal as well as external, and anticipating those that may arise, you can make sure to include solutions to overcome them in your plan. The more you identify your temptations and carry out specific plans for healthier responses, the more you will enjoy peace of mind and once again be in control of your destiny. Here are the pitfalls our client Gayle listed to her goal of losing weight, with five solutions for each:

PAST COMMON PITFALLS TO REACHING A HEALTHY WEIGHT AND FIVE POSSIBLE SOLUTIONS

- Cooking while on weight-loss program
    1. Plan family time over workouts rather than meals.
    2. Let older family members cook for themselves.
    3. Don't taste while cooking.

4. Cook less often or only on Sundays.

5. Cook healthfully for everyone.

- Snacking
    1. Stick to regular mealtimes.
    2. Drink water, chew sugarless gum.
    3. Do something else.
    4. Ask myself if I'm really hungry. (Has it been three or four hours since I last ate?)
    5. Eat only healthful snacks.

- Stress eating
    1. Walk instead.
    2. Breathe deeply.
    3. Take a break at work.
    4. Engage my intellect.
    5. Take a nap.

- Boredom
    1. Read.
    2. Call a friend.
    3. Watch a movie.
    4. Visit family.
    5. Surf the 'Net or daydream.

- No walking partner
    1. Go to fitness center.
    2. Turn on exercise video.
    3. Get a stationary bike.
    4. Walk alone.
    5. Ride bicycle on bike path in park.

Stay Solution-Oriented

Once you start, once you take your first steps, you will soon gain valuable feedback. Both external responses from those around you and an internal response from your spirit will let you know whether the moves you are making are effectively advancing you toward your goal.

What happens if you *do* take a wrong step? Whenever you find yourself facing a difficult situation or crisis, turn your mental processes (mind), physiology (body), and spiritual energy (spirit) into problem-solving mode. First, ask your spirit for guidance and direction by tapping into your intuition, your internal feedback mechanism. What sense or feeling are you getting about the current step? Are you feeling uneasy, uncomfortable, or irritable? You may have a gut sense that the path you've taken just isn't the right one for you. These may be signs to consider an alternate route. Don't forget, though, that you are changing habits that have been with you for most of your life: you are bound to experience some resistance. Sometimes when disciplining the mind and body we will experience discomfort and want to give in. Do not mistake resistance as a sign to quit! Just take note of what and how you feel.

Next, use your mind to get a handle on the nature of the conflict. Is it the timing, planning, or execution of your plan that is making you uneasy? Does your plan lack adequate structure, preventing you from making steady progress? What does your body tell you about your current path? Write down whatever you believe the issue to be.

Now that you have a better understanding of the problem, it's time to switch into "solutions mode." Dr. P always says that there are no problems, only solutions. Rather than hitting your head against the proverbial brick wall or giving up altogether, let yourself relax and look at your situation from another perspective. If the path just isn't working for you, don't force it. Instead, start looking for solutions to your dilemma. See if you can list five possible solutions to address it.

As you look for these means of resolution, you may be led in another direction altogether. If this happens, consider it an adventure! That's what alive and healthy people do. Take in stride any feedback or correction you receive and move on with an attitude of playfulness and optimism. Don't be frustrated or disappointed by the change in your plans: that would only be putting forth additional energy in the wrong direction. Instead, rejoice that your plan has evolved—as all the best plans do!—and move forward with renewed enthusiasm. When you adopt this attitude, you cannot be beaten. Stick to your visualization of the goal and trust that your journey *will* lead you there. You know that your outlook and perception can be directed by your mind, so keep your optimism high. You could even pretend that the new direction was what you intended in the first place. Perhaps it was!

*I will explore various pathways
to my health goal.*

I will set realistic time lines for myself.

I will:
- *deprogram my life of destructive behaviors.*
- *reprogram my mind and body to crave healthy activities.*
- *foresee potential pitfalls and address them ahead of time.*

If I encounter a problem, I will switch into "solutions mode" and go where it leads me with renewed enthusiasm.

CHAPTER 9

Step 4: Chart Your Progress

You have a goal that will transform your life for the better. You have a plan to integrate your spirit, mind, and body. You know where you're going and how you plan to get there. You also know that the journey will take time. Your mind knows this, and yet something inside you wants to see progress right away. When we finally commit to a plan like this, it's because *we want this goal so much*—how can we not be impatient? Yet you won't reach your health goals overnight, just as you didn't get into your current condition overnight. To fight discouragement and keep your motivation high, the fourth step of the plan asks you to track your progress on your journey toward wellness.

Make a daily practice of writing in your journal about the things you experience as you put your plan into motion. If you're not the type to keep a detailed diary, at least make little notes of your successes on a calendar so that you can track how far you've come. Summarize each day's noteworthy events. Take note of things you did, ways you behaved, and how others responded to you. Pay particular attention to strong emotions you experienced along the way, whether they are sadness, anxiety, discouragement or depression, or happiness, confidence, and increased determination. What was it that made you feel that way? As you find emotions or behaviors shifting, write that down to document your progress. Each time you achieve a milestone or see significant improvements, make note of it. Are you finding that certain old habits feel less comfortable? Begin writing these things down each day in a journal and many insights will be revealed to you. Your progress may seem subtle or even unnoticeable to you at first, but when you review the journal in a few weeks, you'll find that a dramatic transformation has begun.

Self-monitoring, as this technique is called, is crucial to your attainment of the goal: it is the cornerstone of most self-improvement programs. Clinical studies have shown that when people monitor their eating habits and exercise activity, their success rates jump dramatically. Journaling to keep track of their progress also gives them satisfaction and significant encouragement. Self-monitoring proves your own power for change. We tend to define "success" as the complete transformation of our health, but in making this assumption we devalue the journey we take to get there. Journaling asks you to pay attention to the individual steps you are taking on your way to success. Noting your behaviors and successes in a diary is itself reinforcing and motivating. When you observe the small changes you make, you find that they, too, are truly dramatic improvements. You gain a deeper appreciation of how each step adds to the profound remodeling process that is taking place.

Self-monitoring also helps you keep track of the behaviors that might be holding you back or limiting your progress. Because we rarely monitor our own activities methodically, many of us are unaware of the extent to which we engage in certain behaviors. If these habits are destructive in any way, they can cause *dis*-ease or block our progress without us even realizing that this is going on. To change your behaviors effectively, you must be aware of the behaviors you need to change: a journal reminds you of them and allows you to track your responses, good and bad, each step along the way. Keeping a journal will also help you remember the strategies you develop to overcome obstacles, which can provide you with answers to future problems that arise. You may even choose to share your notes with others who ask how you made such amazing progress, which, if you follow this plan with diligence, you will.

Review the notes in your journal once a month—more often if you're not satisfied with the progress you're making, so as to identify possible sources of your difficulty. This review can be enormously stimulating and encouraging.

Elsie's Story

Elsie, a lawyer who suffered from arthritis and came to us for weight management, was surprised to discover in her journal a power she never knew she had to overcome the habits and thought processes that once trapped her.

Elsie at first looked at exercise as a tedious chore. She regarded staying on the couch, pandering to her taste buds, and giving in to cravings as her personal right and privilege. She thought we were nuts to insist that food should not be relied upon for comfort or stress relief. Years of being overweight had also given Elsie an oppressively low opinion of her own self-worth. She just didn't believe she could lose weight, it was as simple as that. She scoffed at our belief that she *did* have the power to take control over her eating habits and change her mindset.

Yet Elsie followed our instructions, listing solutions to employ when she felt tempted to give in to negativity, inactivity, and comfort-eating; following her plan; and describing the results in her journal.

She slowly started losing weight. She noticed a gradual lightening in her mood. Then, reviewing her notes one afternoon, she noticed that greater and deeper changes were taking place as well. Elsie had believed that by opting for inactivity over exercise, she was expressing her free will and power to choose. Reflecting on her journal entries, she understood that in the past she had been controlled and manipulated by her ego to believe that she was in control, when in actuality she was driven by subconscious messages of fear. She had admitted in her journal that, as the only woman in her law office, she was afraid of attracting even more attention from the men. She worried that if she did slim down and get more attractive, she would have even less chance of being regarded as smart and competent. Her early notes reminded her, too, of how hard it was at first to resist her contempt for the plan and for herself. Her diary showed that in less than a month she got over hurdles of inertia and found herself doing things she would have never dreamed possible. Most notably, in a matter of weeks she was exercising regularly—and loving it. She looked at food differently and gained more control of her emotions.

Elsie was astonished to find that she really did prefer activity over a sedentary life, both for the overall health of her body and, most important, for her achy joints. She started going out with friends again and doing things she had enjoyed before her body had begun to ache so terribly. Reading through her journal was like a revelation: she had gained control over her eating habits and her mind; she had taken true control of her life and was taking steps toward living it to the fullest.

So take note of the progress you make and be energized by it. The sense of satisfaction you get will inspire you to carry on in your journey. You will prove to yourself that you can accomplish anything you set your mind to. Anytime you think you're not seeing results, read your journal to confirm your accomplishments. Keeping track of your advancement will reinforce the belief that you have the power to change your life for the better. If you become discouraged, you can always return to this book for a gentle nudge back onto the path, but your personal notes will describe your own efforts best. Once you prove to yourself that you can gain little victories, the "big win" will come even easier.

So prove it to yourself by following the plan for thirty days, recording your experiences in your journal, and reviewing it periodically. That's the challenge we gave to Joel, who visited the Institute for anger management. Joel came from a family where rage was the norm. If people didn't do things his way or couldn't understand his point of view, he would explode, cursing and often threatening them. This made all of his interpersonal relationships very trying and painful, and his road rage got him into frequent confrontations and even fights. Joel thought that controlling his temper would be the hardest thing he'd ever do in life—if he ever did it at all. He admitted that he couldn't see how any motivational plan could alter his anger. But Joel had good reasons to attempt this change. He wanted to be a better father to his daughter, Angel, and he wanted to save his marriage to his wife, Alice. He promised to attempt the thirty-day mental diet and complete all five steps of the plan during that month. He agreed to visualize himself as more calm, understanding, and patient, and to follow his progress in a journal.

Joel was lucky to have a business partner, Pete, who embodied the qualities he sought to embrace. He took note of what Pete did in bothersome situations and came up with these five paths toward a more peaceful, even-tempered disposition.

Before flying off the handle at someone, I will:

1. Consider the person a friend, relative, or foreign diplomat. (Pete often imagines people to be the Dalai Lama.)

2. Take five deep breaths before acting—*not* reacting.

3. Consider how the other person will feel if I explode at them.

4. Get rid of my anger through sports, exercise, or writing.

5. If I still need to communicate anger or frustration, I will do so with a smile. (Pete says that softens his delivery and helps the other guy not to feel attacked.)

After three weeks, Joel skimmed over his journal and found that he was really doing well. As he read his notes about doing the things on his list, he was truly impressed. During a counseling session with Dr. P, he remarked that showing compassion for others got them to accept him more in turn. His own journal says it best:

Other people seem nicer since I changed my way of doing things. People are treating me just the way I wanted my "well self" to be treated. Angel comes to me now for help with her homework, and Alice is spending more time with me as well. Being so angry really pushed people away. I'm starting to let go of it now, and doing more things from my list of goals. I feel like this is working. I'm learning to give more, I guess, and I'm getting more in return. And that sure does make me feel happier.

To further demonstrate how charting your progress fits into the Pennington Plan as a whole, here is an extended excerpt from the journal of Phillip, a client who came to us for help in ending his alcohol addiction.

Goal

My goal is to stop drinking alcohol, forever. I want to stop using alcohol as a crutch for my emotional and financial problems. I want to put an end to the terrible problems it's causing my family and take back control of my life.

What is my "well self" like? Well—my well self will not drink when I get frustrated or annoyed, whether that's at work, paying bills, or any other problem, no matter how tempted I am. My well self will be more optimistic when it comes to things like this. I'll be more focused. My well self will have more fun with my family, and I'll get support from other AA members. I'm going to find new friends (who don't drink) and do new things.

I can imagine myself being more patient and more sure of myself, too. People are talking and we're having fun without alcohol around at all. If I don't drink I'll eat better and exercise more, and that will make me feel stronger.

Motivations

1. I am motivated by my family. I will stick to my plan because I want to show my daughter that she can also overcome financial problems and emotional problems without putting drugs in her body. I don't want Suzy to have a drunk for a father. I don't want her to be ashamed of me.

2. I am motivated by my marriage. I love Joanne; she means the world to me. She has stuck by me, she loves me, and I would be an idiot to throw that away. I will *not* let booze ruin my marriage.

3. I am motivated by my health. Drinking has totally wrecked my body, but I got myself in shape in college, and I can do it again.

I've gotten fat and I have no energy and I hate that. I want to feel and look better.

4. I need to straighten out our whole financial picture, too. My drinking has put us in debt. I know it's going to be tough, we may have to pinch some pennies, but we will pay off those credit cards and get our spending under control. I will not have credit card companies running (ruining) my life.

5. I want to have a clear head. I want to be able to help Suzy with her schoolwork. I want Joanne to know she can rely on me to drive our daughter safely to school events—and not forget! I want to remember things like that more—social things, stuff we need around the house, phone numbers. I can't remember anything when I drink, and I want that to change.

Plan

1. I will attend Alcoholics Anonymous regularly.

2. I will stay away from booze *at all times*. I will get all alcohol out of the house. I will stop going to places where alcohol is served.

3. I will ask everyone to support me by not drinking around me, not asking me every time they see me whether I'm sober, and not telling ol' cousin Henry about my plan until I've completely beat it so I don't have to listen to his negative talk.

4. If I feel tempted, I will call on friends and family members and AA members for support. When I'm feeling anxious, I will chew gum, exercise, or pray, but *I will not drink*.

5. I will sign up for acupuncture and counseling treatment programs.

Pitfalls

1. Previously I have blamed my drinking problem on having alcoholism run in my family, pretending there wasn't much I could do about it. Solution: I will avoid blaming this on my family or upbringing and take responsibility for whatever I do.

2. I haven't been able to resist joining the guys for "just a couple of beers." Solution: I will tell anyone who tries to sabotage my plan that alcoholism is a disease and that I know that even *one drink* can make me relapse. I will avoid those people and not go to the bars with them at all.

3. Whenever I thought that I could have alcohol in the house, I ended up drinking again. Solution: I will remove all alcohol from the house and let everybody know they can't bring it into our home.

Progress Log

Wednesday, April 23

My last beer was on Saturday. I've been away from alcohol for four days now and I do not feel any withdrawals, thank God. I do not have any jitters and I've been able to sleep at night. Joanne is being really helpful and supportive and has helped to distract me from thinking too much about tough stuff.

Monday, May 5

Long day at work. My head was hurting today. I took a cold shower in the evening and talked to Matt on the phone. Today wasn't so easy, but I remembered to think on the bright side of this situation—better health, marriage, etc.—and I guess I can be proud of myself for that. I told Matt I was looking forward to feeling in control instead of surrounded by the mess I've made. I felt encouraged that I could actually see some good in myself. I walked on the treadmill for twenty minutes today.

Friday, May 16

AA meeting tonight. Went pretty well. I met an interesting new guy, Bill, who had kind of a different take on things. I told him I realized that I had to stop blaming my family for this. He said true, but being able to look at the cause and effect of my situation—parents and grandparents all alcoholics with lousy marriages—had really convinced me how destructive booze could be. So in that sense Bill said I was lucky! Coming from a guy with experience shaking this thing, I found that really helped me feel less unlucky. Maybe my family was a blessing in disguise.

I think this process is going to get easier. I am getting more energy and focusing more. I made an appointment with the guy at Fleet Bank to discuss cleaning up my credit.

Suzy needed help with her spelling and actually came to me first! Instead of waiting for Joanne to come home. I think she's starting to trust me again. I told her a bedtime story like when she was a little girl and she told me that she loved me. That beats drinking! I will never drink again.

Saturday, May 24

Joanne wanted to celebrate one month of my being sober so we went to her sister's house and had a nice dinner. Everyone said positive things about how I looked. I overheard Suzy telling her cousins that I had worked with her on homework. She seemed so proud that it brought tears to my eyes. Why couldn't I beat this before? She inspires me, she really does. That girl is something else.

I am proud of my progress so far. It'll take time, but I believe the family will forgive me. I hope I can forgive myself for treating them so badly.

Joel's and Phillip's journals reminded them of the subtle changes in their lives. A nice word from somebody, a request for help from your child, a more energetic feeling, a household task you've been dreading accomplished—these things might otherwise go unnoticed and unappreciated, but they are so important. Journaling also helps with the fifth and final step of the Pennington Plan—celebrating!

AFFIRMATIONS

*I will track my progress to prove
my power for change.*

*I will allow my journal to be my confidant
as I make notes of my successes
and/or stumbling blocks.*

*I will release any doubt of my power
or worth by following each step of
my journey in my journal.*

CHAPTER 10

Step 5: Celebrate Your Success

ind a reason to celebrate *every day*. If you're following your plan diligently, successes will follow. Why wait until the end of your journey to celebrate them? Remember, the joy is in the journey. Celebrating, the fifth and most fun step of the plan, is absolutely crucial to success, so don't neglect it: when you reach a milestone, or anything you consider significant, celebrate! Don't wait until you finally make your goal to do your happy dance. Below are some suggested benefits and ways of congratulating yourself that will stimulate you to make the steps of your plan a regular part of your everyday life and bring more joy into the present.

Celebration Will Keep You on Track

Make no mistake: as you slowly retrain your mind and body, you will oftentimes find yourself at a painful point of resistance, a particularly rough patch of terrain. You've lost those first five pounds, but the next five just don't want to budge. Getting up at 6 a.m. to exercise is still the last thing you want to do. You've ditched the "friends" who kept offering you drinks but haven't found others yet. At points like this you may well find yourself wanting to quit. The road ahead just seems too steep, your body and will too weak. *Now*, precisely at this time, you must take a step back, look at how far you've come, and rejoice in the progress you've already made.

I bet that if you were to look back on some of the challenges or problems you've overcome in your life, you would find that you really have racked up some major achievements. Remembering them can certainly give you great satisfaction, but enjoying your achievements *as they occur* can bolster your confidence, stoke your enthusiasm, and add more excitement to your journey. Celebrate right where you are, realizing that now is but a moment in time and that the stage you're in is *temporary*. As long as you stay focused on the goal, you will make it. So rather than thinking about how much further you have to go, enjoy the gains you've made so far. Basking in the glory of your success will keep you energized and motivated. As you embrace and express your joy, you will reinforce the belief that you *can* take control of your thoughts and habits for the ultimate improvement of your life.

Celebration Will Keep You in the Moment

The present is your gift: it is the time over which you have the greatest power and control. Marking milestones as they occur keeps you in the moment. Being committed to your plan is wonderful, but it creates the risk that you'll always be straining ahead to the next success, never stopping to notice where you are. So devote a few minutes of quiet time or meditation to recognizing your progress up to now.

Briefly let go of thoughts about the next step, the rest of the journey, or what lies ahead. Acknowledge the challenges you had to overcome to reach the point you now occupy. Appreciate the contribution of your spirit, mind, and body to the process. Take a moment to recognize the benefits of your hard work and appreciate your efforts.

Treats

You might choose to recognize and reward yourself for significant milestones, or you might celebrate every time that you do any of the new behaviors that you've outlined in your plan. Have you gotten the proper amount of rest, exercise, and healthy nutrition today? Celebrate! Take a quiet walk in the park, award yourself some time to curl up with a new book, make a "play date" with yourself or a friend and go to a restaurant or movie. Little things mean a lot, and they add up, too. Though you have not yet arrived at your destination, you should enjoy the fruits of the seeds that you've planted and are nurturing with every healthy move. So revel in your personal victories. Give gifts to yourself. They do not have to be material gifts: whatever you treasure most in life, lavish a little of it on yourself. Help that positive energy within you keep flowing, propelling you along your journey. Commending your efforts with little rewards and kudos is very much like stoking a fire. It will keep the flame of your motivation high.

One word of caution: unless you have complete self-control, please don't reward yourself with the very vices that caused your *disease* in the first place. If you're trying to lose weight, don't celebrate with Double Stuff Oreos or Häagen Dazs ice cream! Instead, honor yourself with thirty minutes of "me" time—a massage, a hot bath by candlelight, or a joyful happy dance to a favorite CD.

Rewards That Reinforce Your Efforts

One of our clients, Suzanne, found the idea of celebration particularly helpful for maintaining her motivation in her long journey to weight loss. She really took it to heart and found many ways to exalt her changed lifestyle. Part of Suzanne's plan called for her to stop buying sodas and junk food. This really required her to make a significant change in her life; it was not an easy thing for her to do. So to give herself a nonfood reward at the end of a soda- and junk-food-free week, she used the money she saved to buy new clothes. Not only was the money she'd saved its own reward; going to the clothing store and being able to fit into a smaller size gave her intense joy as well. These things helped keep her on track. She would visualize herself in a new outfit while she exercised on the treadmill, which made it even easier to resist wasting money on snacks. Of course, I realize that "retail therapy" can be abused: if splurging on shoes or other clothing would tempt you to charge up a storm or spend money unwisely, then don't do it. In Suzanne's case, though, she enjoyed this treat responsibly: she limited herself to the money she'd saved and knew she could afford. She also involved her nine-year-old daughter, doubling the value of her reward to herself by using it to teach her daughter the importance of saving and budgeting.

Celebrating her success along the way gave Suzanne a renewed sense of confidence and revitalized her self-esteem. The more she got out of the rut of focusing on the negative circumstances of her life and the long road ahead, the more she realized what a capable and strong woman she really was. She recognized that she no longer had to rely on her physical cravings for "guidance"; instead, she could direct the character of her mood and the steps of her life through her own choosing. For the first time, she really felt like the master of her destiny.

Tell Somebody!

Suzanne's perpetual celebration so lifted her spirits that her coworkers began to ask about her new attitude. The "old Suzanne" had shared their views on the focused pursuit of health-related goals. Dieting? Exercise? Ugh. Worse than household chores. Coworkers were dumbfounded to learn that Suzanne's more vibrant looks, springier step, and brighter outlook came from a simple five-step nutrition and exercise plan that she had mapped out herself. Yet they were forced to admit that Suzanne had not only improved her looks and energy, she had altered her very consciousness, and was reaching heights of success they never imagined she—or they—could attain. It got them thinking.

Don't wait for someone to ask you. As you celebrate your little personal victories, share your joy and your insights with someone else! Not only will publicizing your success sharpen your own focus and enthusiasm, you may even inspire those around you to make the lifestyle changes that are important to them. Success is contagious, after all. We're not talking about egotistical boasting: you have every right to be proud of your accomplishments. So don't be shy; share your joy!

Praise Yourself

It may sound silly at first, but honoring yourself with celebration and praise will directly enhance your joy in the journey. There are any numbers of ways to do this, whether heartfelt or humorous. You might be satisfied with just taking a quiet moment to give yourself a mental pat on the back: "Bobby, my friend, you did well this week. As a matter of fact, you totally rocked. Keep up the good work." You might take a more active approach, becoming your own internal cheerleader, something we call "self talk." One of our clients told us that this became one of her favorite ways of rewarding herself. "I used to yell at myself, calling myself an idiot or stupid. When I switched to cheerleader or praise-giver mode, it was such a warm and welcome surprise, like, 'Wow, who's that nice person telling me I'm great?' I hardly recognized myself." Or type up a recognition letter or an elaborate certificate of accomplishment and display it prominently in your home or office, where you'll see it often. It may make you smile; it will certainly remind you of how significant and praiseworthy your efforts are.

Celebrate Detours

Most serious journeys require a willingness to detour and occasionally even to retrace your steps. The aim is not to become fixed on only one pathway to your goal, for if we remain stiff and unyielding, like an oak tree, the storms of life may break us in two. The aim is to become flexible, like a stalk of wheat that bends in the wind and survives. Do not lament the slipups, and don't blame yourself for them. You can't afford to allow negative energy in mind or body to depress you and rob you of your drive. Dr. P always suggests that we learn to look at detours as opportunities for new experiences. Be open and enjoy the ride. Your destination will not change even if your path to it does. The universe may be urging you to take another route to your destination, but you will still get there. The joy, you will discover, *is* in the journey.

Imagine you're driving in your car and find you need to detour around some road construction. You would never make the mistake of believing that the roadwork was your fault. Knowing you would still get to your destination would make it easier to accept that you'd be a bit late. Instead of cursing the construction workers and the city and the orange cones and the heavy machinery—none of which would be the slightest bit affected—you might appreciate that you've learned a new route with lovely scenery, slower but less stressful than your usual route, unless you're in a terrible hurry, that is. But although you certainly want to be focused and goal-oriented with your health plan, you are *not* in a hurry. So there is no reason why a minor setback should destroy your mood. Sing a song to pass the time and accept what is happening. You may find yourself enriched by those detours. This is precisely what happened to one of our clients, Madeleine, when she embraced an open, accepting attitude in the midst of setbacks.

Madeleine's Story

Madeleine was headed to Florida by train when the station announced a several-hour delay due to a switching problem on the tracks. Normally, she told me later, she would have been furious. But this time she was heading for a vacation, and she decided not to waste her energy on being upset. She had left home and work behind, after all, and was making progress on her journey toward much-needed relaxation and self-renewal. She knew she would get to the sunny Florida beaches eventually, so she held on to her happy vacation attitude and walked around the station humming a jazzy tune. As she was perusing the new book releases in a crowded shop, a man beside her began humming along with her. Startled and a bit embarrassed, she looked up with a sheepish grin. The man warmly smiling back at her was so handsome that she blushed.

One thing led to another. He introduced himself, and they went off together to get some food, which they barely touched. Madeleine and Jason spent the next two hours getting to know each other. "I was really angry that my train was delayed," he told her, "but you've made the wait worthwhile." They are now engaged to be married. "If you hadn't explained your view of detours," she told us, "I would have been sitting on a wooden bench pouting and fuming with rage. Now I'm in the happiest relationship of my life! I used to get upset when things didn't go according to my plan, but now I feel that I'm somehow part of a much larger plan than my own. I can finally say that I can 'go with the flow,' knowing I'll achieve my goals at the right time. I get much more peace and fulfillment by embracing *every* experience I find myself in, instead of trying to argue half the time with things I can't control."

Detours don't divert you from life—they *are* life. It's all a matter of perspective. If you keep an open, healthy disposition along your journey, you, too, will be less likely to get derailed, for that derailment is only in your mind. So don't despair if your original path has changed. "When a door slams shut, a window opens," as the saying goes: all we need to do is find the window. It may be that the universe has found a better way of bringing you to your goal, one you may not have planned on but that is just as beneficial, or more so. Keep the faith and press on. Look for five solutions to your situation. Remember, shifting into solutions mode switches your physiology and brain chemistry from frustrated inertia to creative flow. Repeat the steps of the Pennington Plan as often as necessary until success is attained. Look at unexpected circumstances as challenges or puzzles to complete. Choose to adopt an attitude of interest and wonder in the ever changing challenges of life.

My mother was not my only teacher in this; I learned from my father as well. One weekend not long ago I was visiting him in the Ruby Mountains of Nevada. We took a hike along the Ruby Crest and, smiling, he pointed to a mountain in the distance. "That's where I get *my* exercise," he said. Standing miles away, Verdi Mountain looked daunting and downright dangerous to me. To my dad it looked like a playground: he climbs it several times a year. He started pointing out different aspects of the mountain that make the climb both challenging and exhilarating. "Those rocky spots on the right can be really tricky. You always risk twisting your ankle. Once I clear 'em, though, I sure do get a rush. And see those thick evergreens beyond the rocks?" I did. The ground beneath them looked dark and chilly to me. "Hiking through that shady bit is my reward for beating the rocks before it. Farther on, you get a patch of smooth trails that take you to the summit pretty quickly. The views on every side are incredible." On the other side of the mountain, he explained, lies Verdi Lake, a place for quiet fishing and peaceful relaxation that truly makes the climb worth the effort. My father uses mountains as his personal exercise facilities, enjoying the milestones along the way, viewing each challenge as a fun little puzzle to be outwitted. His outlook inspires me to look at every uncomfortable situation from a more creative perspective. So as you move through the peaks and valleys of your life, enjoy the process and celebrate the achievement of your personal milestones as often as you can.

AFFIRMATIONS

I will bask in my accomplishments and celebrate my successes big and small.

I will reward my efforts with special treatment, pampering, and self-praise.

I will congratulate myself for every victory.

I will share my joy with others.

I will celebrate detours as opportunities for new discovery.

I will consider setbacks as mere challenges to overcome.

Applying the Pennington Plan
in Your Life

This five-step plan lays the foundation for the integration of your whole self. We are three-part beings, composed of spirit, mind, and body. Our truest identity, our most innermost self, is spirit: perfect, whole, and infinitely wise. This may be hard to accept, and it is impossible to prove. Certainly as a physician trained in evidence-based medicine, I find it challenging to teach. Nonetheless, it is a concept that resonates with my heart and soul and grants me immense serenity. Believing that on a higher level I am already whole—whatever challenges my body and mind are enduring at the moment—releases me from fear and insecurity and gives me a faith in myself that cannot be shaken. That is why, even though I cannot trap spirit under a microscope to prove to you its validity, identity, and makeup, I believe it to be the most real part of our existence. I have seen intense pain and suffering as people have become trapped in their flesh through wrongly perceiving the physical body as the ultimate self. And I have also seen those who expand their identity from flesh to spirit not only overcome illness but blossom and transform their lives into rich demonstrations of creative beauty. It is certainly much easier to focus upon that which we see, feel, and hear than to pay heed to glimpses and faint whisperings of your spirit, but this is what we must do in order to truly be well and live well.

This plan is but one step on your path to reawakening to your true destiny. Again, this is not a fad diet or a quick fix: the process that you are beginning here will be a lifelong one. Your personal challenge will be to find and embrace your own spiritual truth, then to begin living it. Use this plan to get out of your head and into your heart—to identify and explore your true strengths, potential, and purpose in life. Make the practices you learn in this book part of your daily life. As you record your observations, feelings, and intuitions in your journal, you may begin to sense a guiding force gently ushering you through the peaks and valleys of life—never promising to erase obstacles but offering assistance in rising above them or allowing you to see through them. Trust this part of yourself; it will sustain you while you retrain your mind, body, and spirit to propel you toward better health and vitality.

Life is a journey filled with riveting ups and tumultuous downs. Navigating that journey is challenging. The struggles we face can be discouraging and disheartening, but they can only drag us down if we let them. We *always* have a choice in the matter. Emotional or physical hardships can certainly trip us up temporarily, but they need not permanently prevent us from laughing, loving, and living a full life. It all depends upon where we focus our energies.

Sticking to a new regimen takes dedication. The Pennington Plan offers you a guiding mechanism to help provide structure, direction, and motivation to adhere to any new strategy that you design. But all the plan really does is put the power in your hands. You are, and will always be, the principal architect of your well life. As you apply the plan, remember that you are in control over your thoughts, reactions, and behaviors. You dictate the quality of your life by simply holding on to your convictions and steadfastly moving toward your goals.

Let us briefly review a few suggestions for the successful application of the Pennington Plan, strategies that have helped me, my mother, and many of our patients overcome battles with dis-ease, fatigue, and lack of motivation as we pursue our highest goals and aspirations.

Beware the Comparison Trap

Avoid comparing yourself too harshly with others who already seem to possess the goals you are striving to achieve. The comparison trap can undermine your confidence. Attaining the same result as someone else may cost you more time or effort, but don't become discouraged. You are meant to live *your* life *your* way and in *your* time. You may take strength from the examples of others, but do not take on any pressure to be like them.

Unfortunately, many of us are socialized to believe in conformity. In efforts to garner acceptance and approval, we try to be like those whom we imagine are better than ourselves. Certainly we can be inspired by the example of others, learning from them or taking cues from their behavior—as long as we don't lose ourselves in the process. Remember that we are each unique individuals, born separately, at different times and to different circumstances. We are distinct and precious, and our paths are sprinkled with the opportunities we need to complete our *own* journey. Comparing your successes with those of your neighbor can only hinder your progress. Instead, take that time and energy and channel it into positive thought and action. You do not need to have a body like anyone else, follow the customs of anyone else, or live like anyone else. You need to have the body and habits and life that are right for the innermost *you*. So embrace your uniqueness and live your life for your own enjoyment and development, and for the contribution you can make to the world around you.

Beware the Saboteurs

For any number of reasons, people around you will often try—either consciously or not—to make you doubt you can accomplish your goals. Until others really understand you and how much you are committed to change, even well-meaning friends and family may meddle and interfere. Jealous and insecure people may find it difficult to watch you succeed in the face of their own fears of success. Fortunately, these individuals have *nothing* to do with you.

Don't worry about conforming to the standards of a particular social group unless you truly believe in its values and ideals yourself. When our patients really start to lose a significant amount of weight, for example, so-called friends often tell them they're losing too much or getting too skinny. Of course, in losing weight, as in any other health program, you should see a physician or other health-care provider at least once a year for health evaluations. If your body weight falls well below the national standards for your height and age, then do not dismiss the possibility that you may have an eating disorder. But in the far more likely case that being overweight is subjecting you to health risks that could rob you of your life, tell your friends that you really appreciate their concern and ask that they redirect their support toward the image you seek to embrace—not the image they think is right for you.

Surround yourself with positive, supportive people. Dismiss the advice of naysayers and avoid those who would seek to subvert your efforts at success. Your ability to reach the pinnacle of success was given to you with your first breath of life. It is your right and your heritage. Society, religious customs, friends, and family can only undermine your confidence if you believe what they say. The only way someone else can control your destiny is if you allow them to do so. Of course, the dramatic change you are making in your life will take some getting used to, for yourself and for others. You certainly would not want to alienate friends and family, so give them some time to adjust to your new regimen and way of behaving and to appreciate that you are doing what is best for you. If all else fails, keep your personal dreams and plans to yourself.

Be in the Moment: Accept What Is

No one ever promised us life would be fair. Facing a tragedy like a life-threatening illness is so hard: it may seem as though all the cards are stacked against you. But no matter how much life is left to you, whether days or decades, you have the power to make it something special. Rather than focusing on what could be or should be, choose to act in the present moment. Accept what is and make the most of it. Remember, even as you embrace the moment, that it is still temporary. Learn to savor and celebrate the high points along the way, as they occur. The present is where the action is.

Act, Don't React

Securing a better life for yourself means channeling your energies in healthful ways. Anytime you are faced with a challenge, remember to switch into solutions mode and begin looking for five pathways to help you out of the hole. Rather than burying your head in the sand when life gets rough, stay focused on solutions. You will be amazed at how quickly your burdens will lighten—especially when you actively look for multiple ways to improve your situation.

If you cannot think of what to do next, ask yourself: What would my well self do? Act in the manner that most closely resembles your ideals. We have talked a lot about how a lifetime of subconscious conditioning affects our thoughts and behaviors. Rather than automatically reacting to challenges with stale patterns from the past, engage the fresh, new perspective that you have developed here and choose your thoughts and actions wisely. Similarly, act as much as possible from internal conviction, rather than allowing outside circumstances to dictate your reactions. You always have the power to change your life and path as long as you make conscious choices based on what you ultimately want from life.

You are now armed with the necessary skills to bring your dreams into reality. By employing them, you can raise your mood and your thinking to a higher plane, live with greater vitality, and attain inner peace. Each step is critical to the process. Each step helps to solidify your goal in your mind, to maintain your energy and enthusiasm, and to motivate you to stick with your plan, no matter what. We wish you true wellness. Bon voyage!

INDEX

spirit (*cont.*)
  questions to ask of, 33–35
  quietude of mind, 35, 41, 69
  solitude, 38–39, 86
  in state of wellness, 7–8, 105
  as true self, 18, 26–27
  yoga, 40, 69
strategies for success
  acting in present moment, 176–179, 185
  avoidance of comparisons, 183
  avoidance of unsupportive people, 184–185
  focus on solutions, 156–157, 185–186
strength, exercise for, 95
stress. *See also* lifestyle factors
  burnout, 83–85
  as cause of illness, 78
  high blood pressure, 80–83
  nutritional supplements, 84, 96
  positive function of, 79–80
  rest and relaxation, 86–87
  triggers, 150
subconscious beliefs
  behavioral choices, 16
  concepts and attitudes, 56–60
  influence of, 51–52, 57–60, 68
  memories, 54–56
  reprogramming, 55, 60–63, 148–152
  source of feelings, 63–67
success. *See also* progress, charting of
  celebration of
    affirmations concerning, 180
    benefits of celebration, 171–173
    rewards, 173–174
    self-praise, 175–176
    setbacks and detours, 176–179
  strategies for
    acting in present moment, 176–179, 185
    avoidance of comparisons, 183
    avoidance of unsupportive people, 184–185

focus on solutions, 156–157, 185–186
supplements, nutritional, 84, 96–98

thirty-day mental diet, 71–73, 163
thought patterns
  affirmations concerning, 74
  negative
    influence over illness, 19, 58–60, 68, 72
    overcoming, 11, 60–63, 72, 124–125
    self-defeat, 120
  positive
    in beliefs and actions, 68–70
    optimistic approach to setbacks, 120
    thirty-day mental diet, 71–73, 163
    transcendence of illness, 19–20
subconscious beliefs
  behavioral choices, 16
  concepts and attitudes, 56–60
  influence of, 51–52, 57–60, 68
  memories, 54–56
  reprogramming, 55, 60–63, 148–152
  source of feelings, 63–67
time management for self-nurturing, 86, 109–111
true self. *See* spirit

unsupportive people, 29, 184–185

values, 136–137
visualization
  attainment of goal, 123–125
  motivation through make-believe, 128–132
  of well life, 122–123
  of well self, 118–121, 125–127

wellness
  affirmations concerning, 21
  balance of spirit, mind, body, 8, 11–12, 20

A
Goodfella's
GUIDE TO
NEW YORK